362.1097
Lassite
Multicu

D0287739

Multicultural Clients

Multicultural Clients

A PROFESSIONAL HANDBOOK FOR HEALTH CARE PROVIDERS AND SOCIAL WORKERS

Sybil M. Lassiter

362.10973
L347m

Greenwood Press ———————————————
WESTPORT, CONNECTICUT • LONDON

5/97
CUYAHOGA COMMUNITY COLLEGE
METRO CAMPUS LIBRARY

Library of Congress Cataloging-in-Publication Data

Lassiter, Sybil M.
  Multicultural clients : a professional handbook for health care
providers and social workers / Sybil M. Lassiter.
    p. cm.
  Includes bibliographical references and index.
  ISBN 0–313–29140–3 (alk. paper)
  1. Transcultural medical care—United States. 2. Social work with
minorities—United States. 3. Minorities—United States—Social
life and customs. I. Title.
  RA418.5.T73L37 1995
  362.1'0973—dc20   94–30927

British Library Cataloguing in Publication Data is available.

Copyright © 1995 by Sybil M. Lassiter

All rights reserved. No portion of this book may be
reproduced, by any process or technique, without the
express written consent of the publisher.

Library of Congress Catalog Card Number: 94–30927
ISBN: 0–313–29140–3

First published in 1995

Greenwood Press, 88 Post Road West, Westport, CT 06881
An imprint of Greenwood Publishing Group, Inc.

Printed in the United States of America

∞

The paper used in this book complies with the
Permanent Paper Standard issued by the National
Information Standards Organization (Z39.48–1984).

10 9 8 7 6 5 4 3 2

In memory of my loving parents

Lillian and Aubrey

And to my dear children

**Courtney, Viviene,
and Yasmine**

Contents

Contents

Acknowledgments

I thank those who diligently reviewed and critiqued chapters or served as resources, particularly Saad Ahmed, Srinivasa Rao Patibandla, Cuc Vo Thi Cochran, Linda Nold, Cyndie Smith, Sally Barhydt, Madhavi Ratnaraj, Jayant Rajamani, Pavan Kumar Kamar, Elaine Wittmann, Dorothea Hayes, Erma Bahenburg, and Herfera and Winston Dixon.

Also I sincerely appreciate the dedicated assistance of the librarians at Adelphi University, Carol Schroeder, Victor Oliver, and Marilyn Lesser; and at East Tennessee State University, Marcellus Turner and Martha Earl. Finally, I am indebted to my family, friends, and students who contributed relevant suggestions and offered valued support.

Introduction

Ask not what kind of disease a person has, ask what kind of person has the disease.

—Sir William Osler, 1849–1919

The United States is the most ethnically diverse nation in the world. Its residents represent over 100 ethnic, racial, and cultural groups from every part of the world (Hopkins-Kavanagh & Kennedy, 1992). According to U.S. Census projections, by the middle of the twenty-first century, the average U.S. resident will trace his or her ancestry to Africa, Asia, the Pacific Islands, or the Hispanic or Arab countries rather than to European roots. This theory is known as the "browning of America" (Henry, 1990).

Although the melting pot concept has frequently been ascribed to American society, a more accurate description would be a mixed salad. The melting pot concept tends to ignore the unique qualities that ethnic groups contribute to society by assuming generalized acculturation, the process whereby cultural differences are minimized and ethnic groups adopt the aspects of the majority culture (Fuller & Schaller-Ayers, 1990). That many ethnic groups prefer to maintain their uniqueness is observed in public demonstrations that manifest a sense of pride in their ethnic differences promoting a "we" feeling among their members (Mindel, Haberstein & Wright, 1988). Therefore the mixed salad concept better describes this society, a complementary combination of various elements. Just as the magnificence of nature is attributed to its diversity, so the uniqueness of America is contingent on its diversity.

With any discussion of differing cultures, stereotyping becomes a concern. According to Webster, "a stereotype is an unvarying form or pattern fixed on conventional expression, notion, character, mental pattern, etc., having no individuality as though cast from a mold." In contrast, this book emphasizes that people from any culture should be viewed as individuals who may subscribe to the standards of their culture to varying degrees and in varying situations, or not at all. Throughout the book, the word *some* is used as a reminder that the information presented does not necessarily apply to all individuals of a culture. Notably, there are often more differences in beliefs and practices within cultures than between cultures. By focusing on individual differences, efforts can be made to avoid stereotyping, which often ascribes general negative characteristics to a group. Therefore I invited individuals representing the various cultural groups discussed in the book to critique the chapters. The purpose was to identify and eliminate any content that they felt was offensive or a negative reference to their cultures.

To avoid risking the label *stereotyping* when discussing cultural variations, one alternative is to ignore cultural and individual differences and assume that all people are alike. Most would agree that this approach is unacceptable. The other alternative is to acknowledge cultural differences and manage diversity by developing awareness, sensitivity, knowledge, and skills that encourage effective interactions that are enhanced rather than hindered by differences (Hopkins-Kavanagh & Kennedy, 1992; Pedersen, 1988). This book offers some knowledge about cultures, but awareness, sensitivity, and skills must be developed by the individual health provider.

Culture, broadly defined, is the way of life of a particular group of people (Germain, 1992). Health preservation, prevention, illness, treatment, coping styles, and beliefs about death and dying are parts of the health component of every culture. Health care systems can vary from the highly technological acute care facilities in the United States to the traditional folk systems of many cultures. Folk systems exist even within highly developed societies of the United States. Except for emergencies, it is likely that a large percentage of clients have used their own "hierarchy of illness resort," or process of help-seeking when ill, before seeking professional health care.

Culture influences the meanings of symptoms and consequently the manner in which health problems are treated (Chrisman & Kleinman, 1980). For example, pain appears to be a significant symptom for urban African Americans, Haitians, and Navajos; impotence for Chinese males; gastrointestinal problems for Italian and Mexican Americans; and weight loss and fever for some Hispanic groups (Harwood, 1981). Culture determines illness behavior. Behaviors such as compliance, decision making, self-care, pessimism, and pain tolerance reflect not only an individual's personality but also the person's cultural attitudes. For example, a cultural attitude holding that illness is punishment for sin, or a curse, or an indication of weakness and thereby unmasculine will affect the client's health behavior. Cultural practices also determine which family member makes decisions about a client's treatment. The primary decision maker and caretaker are predetermined roles in some cultures, although these roles may not correspond to mainstream health system role assignment. Also the accepted mainstream goal of self-care may not be expected of the client within some cultures (Hartog & Hartog, 1983).

Cultural ideas related to death and dying can influence behavior as well. The grieving process will be reflected in the behavior of persons from cultures that view death positively as an escape from a life of suffering to rebirth into a better existence or joining honored ancestors. On the other hand, some cultures may hold a negative view of death as punishment for the sins of life. In addition, religious factors can influence coping style and behavior related to pain tolerance and consequently delay the individual's seeking professional treatment. We must also keep in mind that acculturation, generational level, and socioeconomic level will have an impact on the behavior of individuals within any culture. Regardless of cultural affiliation, socioeconomic status, psychological states (stress, worry, and grief), and situational factors (poor housing, homelessness, unemployment, family disorganization) are causative or contributing factors to the illness of individuals (Harwood, 1981).

This book presents basic information for contemplation, further research, and modification to reflect individual differences. Health professionals should be aware that intragroup differences may often exceed intergroup differences. The purpose of the book is to offer a flexible paradigm or an open framework that can serve as a basis for continued expansion of knowledge. Consequently it is not intended to be encyclopedic or to present complete knowledge of the cultures. Cultural changes, intercultural marriages, and individual variations preclude any attempt to become expert in the knowledge of all cultures. The cultures included in the book were selected on the basis of highest population estimates, according to the 1990 U.S. Census, plus cultural groups that have recently migrated in large numbers and about whom knowledge of health beliefs and practices may be limited.

My interest in cultural diversity began many years ago while observing the families residing in a predominantly African-American community of New York. These families represented a variety of cultures within the African-American minority group—individuals from Panama, Nicaragua, Africa, Jamaica, Haiti, India, southern United States, Puerto Rico, Dominican Republic, and Trinidad. Several Native Americans also lived in the community. I noted that culture is not limited to skin color, language spoken, or area of residence in the United States. For instance, black is a color, not a culture; Hispanic relates to persons whose native language is Spanish, not a culture; and communities in America are not as culturally homogeneous as they may be in other countries.

My motivation to write about cultural diversity evolved from experiences in several clinical situations with student nurses whose nursing care was hampered by the students' lack of knowledge about clients' cultural beliefs and practices. Recently I received a letter from a former student who had graduated and was employed at a major metropolitan hospital in New York City. She stated that although she had received an excellent training in manual nursing skills, she was totally unprepared to deal with the complex responses to illness by individuals of the various cultures encountered in the city. Thus her work experiences after graduation provided a valuable supplement to her education. She was writing to me not to complain or criticize the nursing program but to request that I alert the faculty to the importance of including cultural diversity content in the nursing curriculum. I too believe that information about cultures is crucial to effective assessments and interventions for all health care providers.

The ethnocentrism of the mainstream culture of health providers may offer some security, status, and support to in-group members but may unfortunately result in stigmatization of out-group members. Health professionals, predominantly from white, middle-class backgrounds, must make themselves aware of the basic beliefs and health-related behaviors of other cultural group members (Germain, 1992). This book is intended for use by professional care providers, individuals with special expertise to provide health care services and assistance to clients: nurses, physicians, psychologists, social workers, nutritionists/ dieticians, and various therapists (ANA, 1991).

FORMAT OF THE BOOK

Each chapter discusses a specific cultural group and presents information on a number of areas: population in the United States; communication; socioeconomic status; chief complaint; family; elderly, child rearing; socialization patterns; religious beliefs and practices; culturally based health beliefs and practices; cultural dietary patterns, morbidity and mortality; beliefs about death and dying; and physical assessment. Although modern members of various cultures do not ascribe to most traditional beliefs and practices, they are presented in this book because many individuals feel that tradition is the essence of their culture and thus demonstrates their uniqueness.

REFERENCES

ANA (1991). Standards of clinical nursing practice. *American Nurses Association Publication*, p. 8.

Chrisman, N., & Kleinman, A. (1980). Health beliefs and practices. In Stephan Thernstrom (Ed.), *Harvard Encyclopedia of American Ethnic Groups* (pp. 452–61). Cambridge: Belknap Press of Harvard University Press.

Fuller, J., & Schaller-Ayers, J. (1990). *Health assessment: A nursing approach*. Philadelphia: J. B. Lippincott Co.

Germain, C. (1992). Cultural care: A bridge between sickness, illness, and disease. *Holistic Nurse Practitioner*, 6(3), 1–9.

Hartog, J., & Hartog, E. (1983). Cultural aspects of health and illness behavior in hospitals. *Western Journal of Medicine*, 139(6), 910–16.

Harwood, A. (1981). *Ethnicity and medical care*. Cambridge: Harvard University Press.

Henry, W. A. (1990, April 9). Beyond the melting pot. *Time*, pp. 28–31.

Hopkins-Kavanagh, K., & Kennedy, P. (1992). *Promoting cultural diversity: Strategies for health care professionals.* Newbury Park, CA: Sage Publications.

Mindel, C. H., Haberstein, R. W., & Wright, R., Jr. (1988). *Ethnic families in America: Patterns and variations* (3d ed.). New York: Elsevier.

Pedersen, P. (1988). The three stages of multicultural development: Awareness, knowledge, and skill. In P. Pedersen (Ed.), *A handbook for developing multicultural awareness* (pp. 3–18). Alexandria, VA: American Association for Counseling and Development.

APPENDIX: FOR FURTHER INFORMATION

Readers will find the following general resources useful starting points for their own research.

Periodicals

Journal of Cultural Diversity
5823 Queens Cove
Lisle, IL 60532
(708) 969–3809

The Ethnic Reporter
Published by the National Association for Ethnic Studies (see address under associations)

Spectrum
Published by Unity and Diversity World Council (see address under associations)

Associations and Agencies

Health and Medical

American Healing Association (Alternative Medicine)
811 Ridge Dr.
Glendale, CA 91206

International Academy of Health Professionals
70 Glen Cove Rd., Ste. 209
Roslyn Hts., NY 11577
(516) 621–0620

International Patient Education Council
(Health Services)
P. O. Box 1438
Rockville, MD 20849
(301) 948–1863

American Medical Association (AMA)
515 N. State St.
Chicago, IL 60610
(312) 464–4818

American Nurse's Association (ANA)
600 Maryland Ave. S.W., Ste. 100W
Washington, DC 20024–2571
(202) 554–4444

American Public Health Association
1015 15th St. N.W.
Washington, DC 20005
(202) 789–5600

Social Welfare

American Community Cultural
Center Association
19 Foothills Dr.
Pompton Plains, NJ 07444
(201) 835–2661

Association of Multi-Ethnic Americans
P. O. Box 191726
San Francisco, CA 94119–1726
(510) 523–2632

Ethnic Anonymous (Self-Help)
1631 Belmont Ave., No. 107
Seattle, WA 98122
(206) 325–8091

Ethnic Materials and Information
Exchange Round Table
c/o American Library Association
Office for Library Outreach Services
50 E. Huron
Chicago, IL 60611
(312) 280–4295

National Association for Ethnic Studies
Arizona State University
Dept. of English
Tempe, AZ 85287
(602) 965–2197

National Center for Urban Ethnic Affairs
(Community Action)
P. O. Box 20
Cardinal Sta.
Washington, DC 20064
(202) 319–5129

Unity and Diversity World Council
(International Understanding)
1010 South Flower St., Ste. 401
Los Angeles, CA 90015–1428
(213) 742–6832

Interracial-Intercultural Pride
P. O. Box 191752
San Francisco, CA 94119–1752
(415) 399–9111

Multicultural Clients

1

African Americans

POPULATION IN THE UNITED STATES

African Americans comprise 12% of the American population thereby constituting the nation's largest minority group (Bureau of the Census, 1990). Although since 1940, large numbers of African Americans have migrated to the
North and West Coast, the South remains the homeland for over half of this
population, with 59% of their elderly living in the thirteen southern states (Maryland, Virginia, North Carolina, South Carolina, Georgia, Florida, Alabama, Mis-
sissippi, Tennessee, Kentucky, Louisiana, Arkansas, and Texas) (Bureau of the
Census, 1990). Most individuals who moved away in their youth but maintained
close linear ties with consistent interactions among the family generations frequently return to the South to retire (Osborne, 1978).

Generally, black people are of African origin, many of them ancestors of the
slaves brought to this country over three centuries ago (first slaves arrived in
1619). In the United States most African customs were forbidden, but blacks in
the Caribbean and South America, who also experienced slavery and oppression,
were allowed to retain many family and tribal customs (Branch & Paxton, 1976).

There are diversities among African Americans that relate to geographic origins, age, religious values, level of acculturation, intermarriage, and particularly
socioeconomic status. This chapter focuses on the largest group of English-
speaking African Americans in this country—those whose ancestors were
brought here as slaves and who have their roots in the South (a group sometimes
referred to as native African Americans). Since African Americans of southern

descent represent the largest group, most of the findings in the general literature apply to them.

COMMUNICATION

Some African-American clients may withhold information from health professionals in order to test their skill and intelligence, and some will judge the competence of a physician by the immediate success of the first treatment. The client may lose faith and fail to return if the condition continues or worsens. Thus the health professional needs to explain the disease process and course to the client in clear and concise terms (Snow, 1985).

Communication behavior may sometimes differ between African Americans and white individuals. The African communication behavior mode may be "high-keyed, animated, interpersonal, and confrontational." This mode, characteristic of involvement, "is heated, loud, and generates affect." In contrast, the white middle-class mode tends to be relatively low-keyed, dispassionate, impersonal, characteristically cool, and lacking in affect (Kochman, 1981, p. 18). Although Kochman's study speaks of the white middle class, he fails to consider the black middle-class communication mode.

African-American culture apparently permits a degree of freedom of assertion and expression, promoting an ability to manage anger and hostility at a verbal level without losing self-control. Some African Americans believe that the danger of violence exists more when there is limited verbal communication (Kochman, 1981).

Black English uses words and pronunciations that differ from standard English, used by most whites. Other differences include body language, such as moving in closer than the comfort zone for most whites, and direct eye contact when the black individual is talking but looking away when responding. Many African Americans may not use eye cues to indicate whose turn it is to speak; these patterns are often reversed among whites (Hopper, 1993).

SOCIOECONOMIC STATUS

One-third of African Americans live in poverty. Approximately half reside in central cities, in communities typified by poverty, poor schools, unemployment, periodic street violence, and generally high levels of stress (U.S. Department of Health and Human Services, 1990). Many African Americans experience conflicts and stressors related to discrimination. Individuals vary in their perception and internationalization of stressful racial situations, with the perception and appraisal of a stressful event determined by the person's intelligence, education, self-esteem, previous experiences, and coping style (Lassiter, 1987). African Americans show vast differences in coping abilities.

Dodson (1981) noted that socioeconomic level affects the individual's ability to cope or adapt. The higher the socioeconomic status is, the greater is the individual's ability to cope with a hostile society. Socioeconomic status also affects one's self-concept and determines one's sense of powerlessness. Thus, as socioeconomic level increases, so does the individual's self-esteem, with a concomitant decrease in the sense of powerlessness (Dodson, 1981).

CHIEF COMPLAINT

Some African Americans may be embarrassed to reveal information about bleeding and/or discharges from "private" parts of the body. Traditionally a "cold" could refer to any mucus, not just upper respiratory infections. The expression "cold" can be used to describe pain or increased mucoid secretions from any orifice of the body; for example, cystitis might be called a "cold" of the bladder.

FAMILY

In African societies, survival of the tribe was paramount, and kinship bonds directed tribal life. The philosophy of Africentricity, which fostered communality rather than individuality, permeated the black family in Africa and later in America. In spite of extreme difficulties, American slaves tried to maintain their bonds of family and kinship. Although the demands of urban life-styles have resulted in the adoption of an apparent nuclear family model by 60% of African Americans, the extended family concept maintains a significant influence on the behaviors of many black individuals (Staples, 1988).

The typical African-American family is an extended kinship network extending over wide geographic areas (Staples, 1988). After completing a field study of southern African-American families, Kennedy (1980) described these families as a complex pattern of relationships among a wide range of people, who may or may not be related by birth or marriage. Therefore African-American genograms often do not conform to bloodlines because of the practice of informal adoptions.

The major adaptive strengths of the African-American family are strong kinship bonds and flexibility of family roles. African-American couples are usually more egalitarian with respect to family roles than other couples in mainstream America (Hines & Boyd-Franklin, 1982; Staples, 1988).

The philosophy of the extended family is based on a sense of obligation. When family members are unable to survive alone, they depend on relatives (kin) for support. Martin and Martin (1978), who interviewed members of 30 extended families of small towns and urban areas of southern communities, noted the following characteristics:

• Members depend on each other for emotional, social, and material support. In contrast, the nuclear family reflects not this interdependence but independence and individualism and most frequently is economically independent of relatives.

- The typical household consists of at least four generations. The nuclear family usually encompasses only two generations.

- A dominant family figure keeps the family together, and all members look to this person for leadership. That a female is the dominant figure does not necessarily mean a matriarchal household, however; several male relatives may be highly influential in the decision making. Uncles, cousins, brothers, boyfriends, and "big daddies" may serve as decision makers and father figures to children.

- Reaching across geographic boundaries, family members do not have to live in the base household to be active participants of family activities. The base household is the home of the dominant figure and is the most stable unit of the family network. This base is usually the site for family reunions, vacations, holiday celebrations, and other important family activities.

- The family has a built-in mutual aid system for providing aid and moral support to family members. For example, an elderly member who is no longer able to live alone will be taken in by another family member, and children will be cared for ("child keeping") when necessary by any other member, without the technicalities of legal adoption.

- The subextended family may resemble the nuclear family since it is a separate household consisting of a husband, wife, and children. Nevertheless, it is firmly rooted in the base household and is obligated to assist in any family crisis. A family with an absent father may be viewed by mainstream culture as a broken home or a dysfunctional family, but in reality, this family may be an important link in the flexible extended family network with a strong support system (Martin & Martin, 1978).

- Adult children are expected to perform duties for their parents as reciprocal acts. The basic idea of reciprocity is "give and take" and "what goes around, comes around" (Hines & Boyd-Franklin, 1982).

Unlike many white families that were patriarchies maintained by the economic dependence of women, African-American couples have been characteristically more egalitarian in their roles, partly because the system of slavery in the United States did not allow the black male to assume a superior role in the family and the female was not economically dependent on him. Therefore, relationships between the sexes were based on social-psychological factors rather than on an economic compulsion to marry and remain married. This may be an important factor projected into the current philosophy of some African American male-female relationships (Staples, 1988).

One problem faced particularly by African Americans is the imbalanced sex ratio, which places African-American women in competition for the limited number of available men. Often the men for whom they compete are married and not available, a situation that places extreme pressure on the marriages of some African Americans (Staples, 1988).

Another consideration is that African-American women are generally better educated than the men at all levels except the doctoral level. Women tend to have more positions in the expanding sectors of the economy, whereas men are overrepresented in the decreasing number of industrial jobs. Nevertheless, many African Americans experience well-functioning marriages, with loving and dedicated relationships with their spouses and families. Unfortunately, little research exists on positive marital adjustment, happiness, and satisfaction among African Americans (Staples, 1988).

ELDERLY

Hill (1977) found that African-American elderly were more likely than Caucasian elderly to describe themselves as "happy" with few problems adjusting to aging. Perhaps one of the reasons is that they often continue to play an important role in the extended family for advice and child care. Only 4% of African-American families have dependent elders 65 years of age or older living with them. Instead the elder (usually a grandmother) takes young children into her household. Because of this common practice, many African-American families are headed by an elderly woman, caring for dependent children who are not her offspring (Hill, 1977; Staples, 1988).

Although statistics show that generally most whites live longer than blacks, African-American elderly, male and female, who live to be 70 to 75 years or older, have longer life expectancies than their white counterparts (Watson, 1990). This is known as the black/white mortality crossover: there is a lower white mortality rate at younger ages but lower black rates at older ages (Wing, Manton, Stallard, Hames & Tryoler, 1985).

CHILD REARING

Fertility rates of African Americans are related to socioeconomic status and regional characteristics. The birth rate of college-educated African-American women is lower than that of their white counterparts (Staples, 1988). In a study on abortions, Cummings (1983) found that 26% of black women had abortions as compared to 41% of white women. Attitudes about abortion were investigated by Secret (1987), who found that "Southern blacks on the average, approve of abortions less than do Northern blacks and that Southern blacks approve of abortion less than whites" (p. 360). Thus African-American women in the South have tended to seek abortions less often than women in the North and less often than white women in general. Wattleton (1992) noted that when abortion was illegal, affluent women (usually white women) were better able to circumvent the law. However, even assessibility to birth control methods and legalization of abortion have not guaranteed access to these services for less affluent African Americans. Because of inadequate contraceptive usage, African-American women are twice as likely as white women to experience unplanned pregnancies.

Although some African-American women describe menstruation as being "sick," pregnancy is viewed as a state of wellness. Sexual relations are thus considered natural during pregnancy. African-American men see their women as most beautiful during pregnancy and view the pregnancy as a positive sign of their virility and masculinity. Since pregnancy has been a symbol of fertility, an old practice was to take the pregnant women to the fields and have them plant potatoes and onions. It was believed that this practice would ensure a good crop for the farmer.

Another old southern belief ("old wives tale") was that to promote a successful outcome of pregnancy, the expectant mother should sweep around her bed with a broom (to sweep away evil demons) and then place the broom in her bed. She might encircle the bed with mustard seeds as well to discourage demons. Sometimes an empty bottle would be placed at the bedside overnight. If on the next day a bug was found in the bottle, it was believed to be a trapped demon (Carrington, 1978). Other old wives' tales relate to activity restrictions for the pregnant mother: she should not have her picture taken during pregnancy, for this could cause a stillbirth; she should not reach up with hands above her head, for this might cause the baby to be strangled by the umbilical cord; an unsatisfied craving for a food during pregnancy would cause the baby to be marked (birthmarks on the infant are believed to resemble an item of food craved by the mother during pregnancy) (Carrington, 1978).

Traditionally, it was believed that most maternal cravings were for nourishing foods, but some cravings proved detrimental. Pregnant slaves craved and were given clay ("geophagy") or dirt to eat. Later in many southern and some northern areas, pregnant women craved and ate Argo starch ("pica") instead. It was believed that these substances helped produce a fat baby ("fat" meant "healthy"). Apparently anemic mothers had a greater craving for this starch, but the more starch they ate, the more severe the anemia became, which further increased the craving (Spector, 1979). Pica became such a problem that Gerald Deas, an African-American physician in New York, successfully petitioned Argo to stop producing its starch in large, candy-like lumps that were convenient to eat; this starch is now marketed in powder form. Dr. Deas informed his patients and the community about the dangers of pica.

During labor and delivery, many African-American mothers behave in a stoic, nonhysterical manner. This behavior may be related to their childhood, when emphasis was placed on "proper behavior." Outcries made are usually of a religious nature, such as, "Lord have mercy" or "Help me Jesus." Sometimes outcries call for the woman's own mother. "Granny" midwives (older women skilled in the art of delivery) encouraged the mothers to pray during labor.

Shortly after birth, the parents examine the infant for abnormalities as well as any birthmarks. The ears and joints are examined for an indication of the coloring that the child will have as an adult, since the melanin that provides color to African Americans is not completely formed or evenly distributed at birth.

Naming the child confirms the child with an identity. Black Muslim fathers may name the baby, informing the mother of the name later, but most parents cooperate in the naming process. Names are frequently selected from the Bible, or babies are often named after members of the extended family. Recently, black parents have been selecting names of African origin, such as Faraja ("leader of the way") or Turmani ("our trust and hope") (Greathouse & Miller, 1981).

Infant feeding varies depending on socioeconomic status, the need for the mother to return to work outside the home, and religious practices. Most Black Muslim mothers prefer to breast-feed. Many African-American mothers tend to introduce solid foods into the infant's diet earlier than usual (Greathouse & Miller, 1981).

If parents feel that the infant may have or may develop an umbilical hernia from crying or straining at bowel movements, they may strap a fifty-cent coin to the umbilicus or use a belly band on the infant. Mothers usually remove such devices before taking the baby to the health professional (Carrington, 1978).

Circumcision has become a common practice among African Americans. In the past and in many rural areas where babies were delivered by "Granny" midwives, boys were not generally circumcised, but now that most births occur in hospitals, the procedure is usually performed before the infant is discharged (Greathouse & Miller, 1981).

African-American mothers tend to start toilet training early and wean their babies from the bottle early. The toilet-trained and weaned child will be easier for the working mother to place in a child care facility. Sometimes the training and weaning from the bottle and pacifier (if used at all) represent a form of early discipline.

With respect to discipline, middle-class families tend to be more liberal and less authoritarian with their children than lower-income families. Spankings are a part of the discipline process and are not considered child abuse. Lower socioeconomic parents generally tend to use more physical punishment (spankings) to deal with improper behavior than do middle- and upper-class parents (Greathouse & Miller, 1981). Although African-American parents are more likely than their white counterparts to use physical rather than verbal punishment, this form of discipline is often tempered by the love most African Americans express for their children (Staples, 1988).

A popular image of the African-American woman is that of "Mammy," the affectionate nursemaid of both white and black children. This image has some basis because historically motherhood has been an important role for the black woman—even more meaningful than the role of wife (Bell, 1971).

Some studies have associated the African-American child with low self-esteem; others have found that these children are not usually likely to suffer from low self-esteem because of many supportive influences: religion, reference groups, group identification, and positive experiences in the extended family (Staples, 1988). Children build self-esteem based on the appraisal and reinforcement from their significant others (Videbeck, 1960). More recent research findings note that low self-esteem was not found among African-American adolescents because these youngsters focused more on the perceived judgments of family members and other significant others than on the opinions of society (Verkuyten, 1988).

SOCIALIZATION PATTERNS

African-American families usually teach their children to develop pride in their race and culture and try to prepare them to cope with racism. The child is taught to function in two different societies, black society and white mainstream society, while maintaining his or her identity and self-esteem. Thus, African-American parents' child-rearing techniques are geared to prepare their children for a kind of existence that may be alien to middle-class white children (Staples, 1988).

Because of the role flexibility in child rearing and household responsibilities within the family, the child may not internalize rigid distinctions between male and female roles. Results of studies comparing African-American and white children indicated that the African-American children were more androgynous, displaying a less stereotypic concept of sex roles than white children (Johnson, 1977; Kleinke & Nicholson, 1979).

CULTURALLY BASED HEALTH BELIEFS AND PRACTICES

Although a number of investigators (Baker & Cook, 1983; Hopper, 1993; Lassiter, 1987; Snow, 1983, 1985; Wilson-Ford, 1992) have identified common health beliefs and practices among many African Americans, these beliefs and practices do not refer to all African Americans. Rather, beliefs about health and related practices vary depending on the degree of adherence to traditional ideas, geographic location, education, scientific orientation, and socioeconomic status. Nevertheless, the Africentric heritage has caused most African Americans to retain a holistic philosophy of health, perceiving mind and body as inseparable and the total person in interaction with the environment. Consequently, many believe that life events affect all aspects of life, including one's job, one's family, and one's health (Snow, 1979). Thus, illness is thought to result from disharmony or conflicts in some area of a person's life (Cherry & Newman-Giger, 1991).

Snow (1983, 1985) led extensive public health studies of low-income blacks. Although he acknowledged the existence of differing black nationalities—Haitian, West Indian, and African American—his study concentrated on the last group, still difficult because of the number of intermarriages, resulting in a blending of many cultural beliefs. Generally, his findings were as follows:

• Some African Americans believe in a twofold classification for the causes of illness, natural or unnatural, with the designation determining where the individual will seek health care. The unnatural causes are due to forces like "worriation" (worry), everyday stress, evil influences, or sorcery. Thus, some believe that hypertension results from stress related to racism and that diabetes is a result of "worriation."

- Some individuals believe that natural illnesses result from an individual's lack of responsibility for protecting himself or herself against illness. Prevention should include avoiding excess heat or cold, eating a healthy diet, and/or keeping the system clean through the regular use of laxatives. Some believe that the failure to worship God through prayer or church attendance could cause a natural illness.

- Some African Americans believe that a cold environment is a frequent cause of natural illnesses, such as upper respiratory infections, head colds, flu, bronchitis, cystitis, pneumonia, and, in later life, arthritis. For example, some individuals may describe arthritis as a cold in the joints.

- A common belief exists that dirt and impurities are a major cause of natural illness. Some African Americans believe that the main purpose of menstruation is to rid the body of dirty blood. Thus, any interference with the normal blood flow can be cause for concern. This traditional belief may be the reason why some African-American women hold negative views about contraceptive devices that could alter menstrual flow.

- Unnatural illnesses may result from forces such as "worriation," stress of everyday life, evil influences, or witchcraft. A "fix" or "hex" (spell), put on a person through witchcraft, may cause the victim to display abnormal physical or mental behavior. The hex is usually accomplished by adding substances to the victim's food. Thus, African Americans who believe in witchcraft are extremely careful about who prepares their food, to the point that some persons will eat only food prepared by self or a close family member.

- Changes in behavior may be the result of a spell, and therefore a folk healer would be the most effective psychotherapist.

- Low-income African Americans use a large variety of home remedies, traditional healing practices, and over-the-counter drugs.

- The use of herbs is a common practice, though noted more in rural than urban areas. Herbs and home remedies are frequently used in conjunction with mainstream professional prescriptions.

- Some African-American clients are suspicious of too many blood tests because blood is a substance that can be used in witchcraft.

- Some fear surgery for cancer, because they believe that exposing cancer cells to air causes its spread.

The results of studies by Lassiter (1987) and Snow (1983, 1985) noted that African-American health practices included the following:

- Health can be maintained by proper nutrition, which means eating three meals a day, including a hot breakfast.

- Laxatives should be used periodically to keep the system open. Castor oil is commonly used.

- Cod liver oil taken especially during the winter months will help prevent colds.

- Copper and silver bracelets worn by young girls through adulthood will protect them during growth. Pending illness will cause the skin around the bracelet to darken, alerting the wearer of a need to change her health habits by improving her diet and/or increasing her rest and prayer periods.

- Women who go swimming or wash their hair while they are menstruating are sometimes more vulnerable to illness.
- Cravings for food, as well as the pregnant woman's thoughts, may affect the health and physical appearance of the baby.
- Home remedies include sugar and turpentine for worms and to cause an abortion; poultices applied to various parts of the body to treat infection and pain; herb teas to treat pain, fever, and gastrointestinal problems; soda to treat chest pain; vinegar and garlic for high blood pressure; and hot tea with lemon and honey and a dash of brandy and/or Vicks Vaporub swallowed to treat a cold.

Wilson-Ford (1992) studied health protective behaviors practiced by 407 elderly black women living in rural North Carolina and identified the following behaviors, listed in order of priority:

1. Eat nutritious food.
2. Pray/believe in God.
3. Use home remedies and over-the-counter drugs.
4. Sleep/rest.
5. Ignore/forget until condition becomes disabling.
6. Reduce stress.
7. Monitor weight and use of salt and sugar.
8. Avoid alcohol and smoking.
9. Contact health care system.

For many African Americans, prayer was expressed as the most common method used for the treatment of illness. Frequently the next move was the "lay referral system"—seeking advice from relatives or significant others. As a final resort, if illness persisted, the professional health care system was consulted (Lassiter, 1987; Snow, 1985).

CULTURAL DIETARY PATTERNS

"Soul food," the expression used to describe African-American food, is preferred by many but certainly not all. During slavery and later, the black plantation worker was often allotted only the undesirable pieces of meat, such as the intestines and bony cuts. Later the ex-slaves purchased their own land and raised pigs and chickens. Consequently, African Americans learned to prepare spareribs (bony part of the pig), chitterlings or "chitlins' " (hog intestines), and pig's feet and ears (interviews with African Americans, 1987). Pork is a popular meat product in the African-American diet. Pork skins, fat, and ham hocks are often used to flavor other dishes. Black Muslims, however, do not eat pork. Other favorite foods that may be included in "soul food" diets are as follows:

- *Vegetables*: collard greens, kale, turnips, corn, sweet potatoes, yams, black-eyed peas, pinto beans, kidney beans, lima beans (butter beans).
- *Cereals and breads*: grits, oatmeal, skillet bread (unleavened corn bread), hoe cake bread (unleavened flour bread), flour dumplings.
- *Dairy*: clabber (similar to yogurt), fried eggs.
- *Meats*: fried chicken, fried pork chops (with gravy), smoked Virginia ham, chitlins', spareribs, scrapple (breakfast meat made from pork scraps), sage sausage, fried fish.
- *Desserts*: rice and bread puddings, homemade biscuits (covered with blackstrap molasses), and various berries (Carrington, 1978).

Seventy-five percent of African Americans do not drink milk because their gastrointestinal tracts cannot tolerate lactose (Boyle & Andrews, 1989). If this problem exists, the health professional can recommend the use of Lactaid tablets or lactose-free milk products available at the supermarket.

Except for individuals who do not eat pork or any other meat products, African Americans generally enjoy foods that are high in fat content and highly seasoned, especially with salt. However, increasing public health information about the adverse effects of fats and salt in relation to heart disease and hypertension has motivated many African Americans to alter their eating habits (DHHS, 1990).

RELIGIOUS BELIEFS AND PRACTICES

Traditionally African Americans have had strong religious orientations. The church was the major institution in the lives of the slaves; its hymns and spirituals communicated ideas about salvation, freedom, judgment and punishment, and plans to escape.

Preachers have always been major speakers among African Americans, and many black politicians and leaders have also been powerful religious figures, among them, Martin Luther King, Jr., Adam Clayton Powell, Malcolm X, and Jesse Jackson (Asante, 1987). The chief purpose of preaching is to stir up the emotions. The church continues to serve many functions in the lives of African Americans, playing an active role in the coping and adaptation processes of its members. The church sponsors activities for the entire family and also provides a network of people who are available as a support system in times of need (Hines & Boyd-Franklin, 1982). African-American churches include Baptist, African Methodist, Episcopal, Jehovah's Witness, Church of God in Christ, Church of Christ, Seventh Day Adventist, Pentecostal, Nation of Islam, Presbyterian, Lutheran, and Roman Catholic (Hines & Boyd-Franklin, 1982).

The largest number of African Americans in the South are Baptists. The Baptist religion began in Switzerland and was brought to this country by the Pilgrims (Wood, 1978). By the middle of the twentieth century, the Baptist religion became the largest Protestant denomination in the United States for both black and white (Gausted, 1987). Baptists stress an individual's personal relationship with God and seek to follow Jesus Christ as He is described in the Bible. Baptists emphasize the individual and attempt to apply their faith to daily life. They believe that the New Testament associates baptism with faith in Jesus; thus, baptism is withheld until individuals can make their own decisions and commitments. According to the New Testament, baptism is synonymous with death and resurrection, cleansing individuals of one way of life so that they can begin a new quality of life as Christians. Most Baptist churches have a baptistery in the floor, a pool of water about waist deep where believers are baptized by immersion (Wood, 1978).

Many African Americans are Methodists, a Protestant denomination that began as a group within the Church of England. The name *Methodist* arose from the description of a follower as a person who lives according to the method laid down in the Bible (Baker, 1987). The early Methodists practiced a methodical daily schedule of duties, visiting the sick and imprisoned, conducting schools for the poor, and praying silently every hour and aloud three times a day (Sockman & Washburn, 1975). The Salvation Army was founded by a Methodist minister, William Booth (Bates, 1977). Methodists teach how to live a Christian life and communicate directly with God. They believe in infant baptism by sprinkling water on the infant's forehead. Methodists view the infant as a member of the church from birth and believe that the child can later decide whether to continue in the faith by making a committed response in confirmation (Bates, 1977; Wood, 1978).

Jehovah's Witnesses generally oppose the teachings of other religious groups. They often reject modern scientific advances, including medicines, and they refuse transfusions of another person's blood. They oppose abortion, artificial insemination, sterilization, euthanasia, organ donations, and faith healing (Spector, 1990).

Seventh Day Adventists regard Saturday as their Sabbath. They accept the Bible and believe that evidence of salvation will be through keeping the commandments. Many groups refrain from alcohol, coffee, tea, narcotics, and stimulants. Most accept therapeutic abortions, autopsy, organ donations, medications, blood transfusions, and surgical procedures. Euthanasia is not practiced. Most Seventh Day Adventists believe in divine healing and prefer a vegetarian diet (Spector, 1979).

The Nation of Islam represents members of the Islamic faith (Muslims/Moslems) of which there are diverse groups throughout the country. Islam is a way of life based on the concept of brotherhood. For the orthodox, all life is dependent on the will of God (Allah), which one understands by reading the holy book, the Quran (or Koran), and the teachings of the prophet, Muhammad.

This religion directs all activities of life. A strong emphasis is placed on self-discipline, as exemplified by prayer and fasting rituals. Muslims pray five times a day and fast during the entire month of Ramadan, when nourishment may be taken only after sunset. Young children, the elderly, pregnant women, and ill persons are exempt from the Ramadan fast. Family roles are traditional; the husband is the major provider and the spiritual leader. In traditional Muslim centers, the women are isolated. They usually wear veils and a long outer garment called the abba or chador. Muslims do not eat pork or pork products and beans. They do not consume alcoholic beverages or substances that interfere with the ability to think clearly. Thus, alcoholism and drug abuse problems are virtually nonexistent in the Muslim community (Ramsey, 1986).

MORBIDITY AND MORTALITY

Death Rate

Life expectancy for African Americans has lagged behind that for the total American population throughout this century, and since the mid-1980s, the gap has increased. Although the life expectancy has risen to 75 years for the overall population, it has fallen for African Americans from a high of 69.7 in 1984 to 69.4 in 1987 (DHHS, 1990). Southern-born African Americans have the highest mortality rates and western-born the lowest. African Americans born in the Northwest, Midwest, and outside the United States have rates intermediate between those born in the South and West (Greenberg & Schneider, 1992).

African-American infant mortality rate is high. A high percentage of low birth weight accounts for the high death rate of African-American babies. Even the infant mortality rate for normal African-American babies is higher than that for white babies. The major killer from birth to 1 year of age is sudden infant death syndrome (DHHS, 1990; Butler, 1992). Braithwaite and Taylor (1992) noted that significantly more African-American births are high risk; African-American mothers were twice as likely as whites to be 18 or 19 years old, to have less than 12 years of education, and to have had late or no prenatal care.

Health Status

There are varying theories associated with the health status of African Americans. Poor health is attributed to decreased access to health care services, discrimination in the health care system, economics, and health care utilization factors (Byrd, 1990; Russell & Jewell, 1992). Statistics indicate that generally African Americans do not receive enough early, routine, and preventive health care (DHHS, 1990). Although poverty may appear to be an underlying element in the disparity of African Americans' utilization of the professional health services, research has found that when socioeconomic factors were controlled, health status indicators still remained consistently poorer for African Americans than for white Americans (National Center for Health Statistics, 1990). Recent research on African-American elders has suggested that culture and ethnicity have an impact on the health behavior of African Americans and their utilization of professional health services. Major deterrents to the use of health services were found to be assessibility and acceptability (Lassiter, 1994).

Hypertension

Hypertension morbidity and mortality rates are at least three to five times higher in African Americans than in Caucasians (Saunders, 1991). In the United States, African Americans living in rural areas have higher systolic blood pressure levels than their counterparts living in urban areas (Wilson, Hollifield & Grim, 1991). African Americans of lower socioeconomic status experience higher rates of hypertension as compared to their advantaged peers. The incidence, severity, and complications of hypertension increase with decreasing educational achievement. Another study noted that since education is the most common indicator of socioeconomic status, African Americans with a greater number of years of education experience less hypertension than less educated individuals (Sorel, Ragland, Syme & Davis, 1992).

Diabetes

Diabetes is 33 percent more prevalent in African Americans than in Caucasians in the United States. African-American women, especially those who are overweight, experience the highest rates (DHHS, 1990).

Coronary Heart Disease

African Americans experience a high rate of coronary heart disease. The higher prevalence of hypertension, diabetes, cigarette smoking, and obesity contributes to their higher level of coronary heart disease (Curry, 1991). Coronary heart disease has been associated with hostility. A relationship has been found between hostility and health behavior that may provide an explanation for the association between hostility and coronary heart disease (Scherwitz, Perkins, Chesney, Hughes, Sidney & Manolio, 1992). However, when heart disease rates were compared within income levels, African-American levels were lower than those for whites (DHHS, 1990).

Cancer

Although cancer remains a major health problem for African Americans, improvement has been noted. Since 1984, the cancer mortality rate for African Americans has declined 2 percent. Black women are having Pap smears more frequently than women of any other ethnic group. The use of tobacco has decreased much more among African-American adolescents than among their white counterparts. There is evidence also that high cancer mortality and morbidity in African Americans may be related to poverty, limited access to health care, and lack of education (Boring, Squires & Health, 1992).

AIDS

The rate of AIDS among African Americans is more than triple that of whites. The number of AIDS cases associated with intravenous drug abusers is greater for African Americans than for other AIDS victims. Also there are higher rates of heterosexual transmission of the HIV virus and thus transmission from mother to newborn (DHHS, 1990; Selik, Castro & Papaionnou, 1988).

Sickle Cell Anemia

Sickle cell anemia is a disease found predominantly in persons of African origin (Jones, Dunbar & Jirovec, 1982). It is estimated that 8 percent of African Americans carry the sickle cell trait and one in 500 have the disease (Brunner & Suddarth, 1988). In Nigeria more than 30% of the people were found to have the trait. It was believed that people with sickle cell anemia have a 50% chance of dying before their twentieth birthday (Jones, Dunbar & Jirovec, 1982). However, recent improvements in sickle cell health education plus advanced crisis intervention measures have increased the chances for a longer life expectancy. In recent years, some with sickle cell anemia have been known to live into their sixties (Brunner & Suddarth, 1988).

BELIEFS ABOUT DEATH AND DYING

These beliefs are generally determined by the religious affiliation and/or by family conditioning. Many African-American funerals are elaborate and attended by the extended family from within and out of the country. These funerals are often preceded by a wake.

PHYSICAL ASSESSMENT

Several studies have noted more mature and rapid skeletal and motor development in African-American children than in white children, and thus African-American children sit up and crawl earlier. They also appear to develop more refined manual skills through the age of 4.

Perhaps due to hereditary factors, African Americans have significantly fewer dental caries than white Americans. Only Chinese Americans appear to have fewer dental caries than African Americans. However, African Americans tend to have a slightly higher rate of periodontal disease than white Americans. Periodontal disease, which causes little or no discomfort (except for bleeding gums during brushing and later loosening teeth), is usually detected by dental check-ups (Pelton, Dunbar, McMillan, Moller & Wolff, 1969).

It is of interest to note that the hair is not typically kinky. Some African Americans have naturally straight, wavy, or loosely curly hair. Popular styles now include hair that is relaxed or worn in cornrows, especially among the females, although many males wear similar styles. Many males wear their hair natural, although the popularity of the Afro (full and rounded cut) has waned (Greathouse & Miller, 1981).

In order to diagnose abnormal color changes in dark-skinned individuals, one must observe the body areas where melanin and carotene are least concentrated: the sclera, conjunctiva, nail beds, lips, palms, soles of feet, and mucous membranes of the mouth (Sherman & Fields, 1982).

Pallor may appear as a yellowish-brown in brown-skinned individuals but will be indicated by an ashen-gray coloring in dark and black individuals.

Cyanosis, when present in dark-skinned persons, may be best seen in facial skin, around the mouth, the earlobes, and nail beds. Pressure to the nail beds and/or earlobes may be used to determine slow or normal return of color. Slow return of color is indicative of cyanosis (Sherman & Fields, 1982).

Jaundice may be observed as a generalized yellowing of the sclera. The normal yellow pigmentation found in dark individuals tends to be concentrated in the inner and outer canthi of the eyes. In jaundice, the palate may also display a yellowish tint. Additional data, such as clay-colored stools and blood test results, may be needed to confirm the presence of jaundice in dark-skinned individuals (Sherman & Fields, 1982).

REFERENCES

Asante, M. K. (1987). *The Africentric idea.* Philadelphia: Temple University Press.

Baker, A., & Cook, G. S. (1983). Stress, adaptation and the black individual. *Journal of Nursing Education, 22*(6), 237–42.

Baker, F. (1987). Methodists. In Mircea Eliade (Ed.), *The encyclopedia of religion* (Vol. 2) (pp. 493–95). New York: Macmillan.

Bates, J. (1977). *The Methodist church.* New York: Religious Education Press.

Bell, R. (1971). The relative importance of mother and wife roles among Negro lower-class women. In R. Staples (Ed.) *The black family: Essays and studies* (pp. 248–56). Belmont, CA: Wadsworth.

Bennett, L., Jr. (1975). *The shaping of black America.* Chicago: Johnson.

Boring, C., Squires, & Health, C., Jr. (1992). Cancer statistics for African Americans. *CA: Cancer Journal for Clinicians, 42*(2), 1251.

Boyle, J. S., & Andrews, M. M. (1989). *Transcultural concepts in nursing care.* Glenview, IL: Scott, Foresman/Little, Brown.

Braithwaite, R. L., & Taylor, S. E. (1992). *Health issues in the black community.* San Francisco: Jossey-Bass.

Branch, M., & Paxton, P. (1976). *Providing safe nursing care for ethnic people of color.* New York: Appleton-Century-Crofts.

Brunner, L., & Suddarth, D. (1988). *Textbook of medical-surgical nursing* (6th ed.). Philadelphia: Lippincott.

Bureau of the Census. (1990). *Statistical abstract of the United States.* Washington, DC: Government Printing Office.

Butler, O. (1992). The reduction of black infant mortality: An eighteen month evaluation of three Tennessee Black Health Care Task Forces' demonstration projects. *Journal of Health and Social Policy, 3*(4), 59–80.

Byrd, W. (1990). Race, biology and health care: Reassessing a relationship. *Journal of Health Care for the Poor and Underserved, 1*(3), 278–96.

Carrington, B. W. (1978). The Afro-American. In A. L. Clark (Ed.), *Culture, childbearing, health professionals* (pp. 34–52). Philadelphia: F. A. Davis Company.

Cherry, B., & Newman-Giger, J. (1991). Black Americans. In J. Newman-Giger & R. E. Davidhizer (Eds.), *Transcultural nursing: Assessment and intervention* (pp. 147–82). St. Louis: Mosby Year Book.

Cummings, J. (1983, November 20). Break up of black family imperils gains of decades. *New York Times*, p. 1.

Curry, C. (1991). Coronary artery disease in African Americans. *Circulation, 83*(4), 1474–75.

Department of Health and Human Services (DHHS). Public Health Services. (1990). *Healthy people 2000: National health promotion and disease prevention objectives* (DHHS Publication PHS 91–50212). Washington, DC: Government Printing Office.

Dodson, J. (1981). Conceptualizations of black families. In H. P. McAdoo (Ed.), *Black families* (pp. 23–36). Beverly Hills: Sage Publications.

Gaustad, E. (1987). Baptists. In M. Eliade (Ed.). *The encyclopedia of religion* (Vol. 2) (pp. 63–66). New York: Macmillan.

Greathouse, B., & Miller, V. G. (1981). The Black American. In A. L. Clark (Ed.), *Culture childrearing* (pp. 68–95). Philadelphia: F. A. Davis Company.

Greenberg, M., & Schneider, D. (1992). Region of birth and mortality of blacks in the United States. *International Journal of Epidemiology, 21*(2), 324–28.

Hill, R. B. (1977). *Informal adoption among black families.* Washington, DC: National Urban League Research Department.

Hines, P. M., & Boyd-Franklin, N. (1982). Black families. In M. McGoldrick, J. K. Pearce & J. Giordano (Eds.), *Ethnicity and family therapy* (pp. 84–107). New York: Guilford Press.

Hopper, S. V. (1993). The influence of ethnicity on the health of older women. *Clinics of Geriatric Medicine, 9*(1), 231–59.

Johnson, J. (1977). Androgyny and the maternal principle. *School Review, 86*(1), 50–69.

Jones, A., Dunbar, C., & Jirovec, M. (1982). *Medical-surgical nursing.* New York: McGraw-Hill.

Kennedy, T. (1980). *You gotta deal with it: Black family relations in a southern community.* New York: Oxford University Press.

Kleinke, C. L., & Nicholson, T. (1979). Black and white children's awareness of de facto race and sex difference. *Developmental Psychology, 15*(2), 84–86.

Kochman, T. (1981). *Black and white styles in conflict.* Chicago: University of Chicago Press.

Lassiter, S. M. (1987). Coping as a function of culture and socio-economic status for

Afro-Americans and Afro-West Indians. *Journal of the New York State Nurses Association, 18*(3), 18–30.

Lassiter, S. M. (1994). *The relationship of cultural health beliefs and practices to health care seeking behaviors in African American elders: A pilot study.* Unpublished manuscript.

Martin, E. P., & Martin, J. M. (1978). *The black extended family.* Chicago: University of Chicago Press.

National Center for Health Statistics. (1990). Department of Health and Human Services. Hyattsville, MD.

Osborne, O. H. (1978). Aging and the black diaspora: The African, Caribbean, and Afro-American experience. In M. Leininger (Ed.), *Transcultural nursing: Concepts, theories and practices* (pp. 317–33). New York: John Wiley & Sons.

Pelton, W. J., Dunbar, J. B., McMillan, R. S., Moller, P., & Wolff, A. E. (1969). *The epidemiology of oral health.* Cambridge: Harvard University Press.

Ramsey, D. E. (1986). The lifestyles of Afro-American Sunni Moslems in New York City. *Journal of the New York State Nurses Association, 17*(1), 21–30.

Russell, K., & Jewell, N. (1992). Cultural impact of health care access: Challenges for improving the health of African Americans. *Journal of Community Health Nursing, 9*(3), 161–69.

Saunders, E. (1991). Hypertension in African Americans. *Circulation, 84*(3), 1465–67.

Scherwitz, L., Perkins, L., Chesney, M., Hughes, G., Sidney, S., & Manolio, T. (1992). Hostility and health behaviors in young adults: The CARDIA Study. *American Journal of Epidemiology, 136*(2), 136–45.

Secret, P. E. (1987). The impact of region on racial differences in attitudes toward legal abortion. *Journal of Black Studies, 17*(3), 347–69.

Selik, R. M., Castro, K. G., & Papaionnou, M. (1988). Racial/ethnic differences in the risk of AIDS in the United States. *American Journal of Public Health, 78*(12), 1539–44.

Sherman, J. L., Jr., & Fields, S. K. (1982). *Guide to patient evaluation* (4th ed.). Garden City, NY: Medical Examination Publishing Co.

Snow, J. Public Health Group. (1985). *Common health care beliefs and practices of Puerto Ricans, Haitians and low income blacks in New York/New Jersey area.* NHSC/DHHS Region 11, Contract 120–83–0011.

Snow, L. F. (1983). Traditional health beliefs and practices among lower class black Americans. *Western Journal of Medicine, 139*(6), 820–28.

Sockman, R. W., & Washburn, P. A. (1975). What is a Methodist? In L. Rosten (Ed.), *Religions of America: Ferment and faith in an age of crisis* (pp. 170–85). New York: Simon and Schuster.

Sorel, J., Raglan, D. R., Syme, S. L., & Davis, W. B. (1992). Educational status and blood pressure: The Second National Health and Nutrition Examination Survey. *American Journal of Epidemiology, 135*(12), 139–48.

Spector, R. E. (1979, 1991). *Cultural diversity in health and illness.* (2d and 3d eds.) New York: Appleton-Century-Crofts.

Staples, R. (1988). The black American family. In C. H. Mindel, R. W. Haberstein & W. Roosevelt Wright, Jr. (Eds.), *Ethnic families in America: Patterns and variations* (pp. 303–24). New York: Elsevier.

Verkuyten, M. (1988). General self-esteem of adolescents from ethnic minorities in the Netherlands and the reflected appraisal process. *Adolescence, 23*(92), 863–71.

Videbeck, R. (1960). Self-conception and the reactions of others. *Sociometry, 23*, 351–59.

Watson, W. (1990). Family care, economics and health. In Z. Harel, E. A. McKinney & M. Williams (Eds.), *Black aged: Understanding diversity and service needs* (pp. 50–68). Newbury Park, CA: Sage.

Wattleton, F. (1992). Reproduction rights and the challenge for African Americans. In R. Braite & S. E. Taylor (Eds.), *Health issues in the black community* (pp. 301–14). San Francisco: Jossey-Bass.

Wilson, T., Hollifield, L., & Grim, C. (1991). Systolic blood pressure levels in black populations of sub-Sahara Africa, the West Indies, and the United States: A meta-analysis. *Hypertension, 18*(3 Suppl.), 187–91.

Wilson-Ford, V. (1992). Health protective behaviors of rural black elderly women. *Health and Social Work, 17*(1), 28–36.

Wing, S., Manton, K. G., Stallard, E., Hames, C. G., & Tryoler, H. A. (1985). The black/white mortality crossover: Investigation in a community-based study. *Journal of Gerontology, 40*(1), 78–84.

Wood, J. (1978). *The Baptists.* New York: Religious Education Press.

2

Arab Americans

The modern Arab countries lie in the Middle East and stretch from the Atlantic Ocean to the Persian Gulf. The Arab world encompasses Algeria, Bahrain, Egypt, Iraq, Jordan, Kuwait, Lebanon, Libya, Mauritania, Morocco, Oman, Qatar, Saudi Arabia, Sudan, Syria, Tunisia, the United Arab Emirates, and Yemen. About three-quarters of the Arabs live in six countries: Algeria, Iraq, Morocco, Sudan, Syria, and Egypt, which has the largest population (Mansfield, 1990; United Nations, 1992).

The Arab countries are located at the crossroads of major trade routes between the East and the West. The strategic importance of Arab lands was enhanced in the twentieth century when it was noted that this area contained the world's largest oil reserves.

The Arab world, encompassing 46 million square miles, is about 25% larger than the United States. The largest country, Sudan, is more than three times the area of Texas, and the smallest, Bahrain, is almost the size of New York City. Although there is a small percentage of Jews and Christians, 94% of the people in the Middle East are Muslim (Lamb, 1987).

POPULATION IN THE UNITED STATES

Although most Arab Americans are descendants of Syrian immigrants, all of the Arab countries are represented in the Arab-American population, including many immigrants who are from Palestine, now the state of Israel (Mansfield, 1990; Naff, 1980).

It is difficult to estimate the number of Arabs in the United States because they are from different countries of origin. Middle Eastern immigrants identify themselves not only in terms of country of origin but by religion, cultural heritage, city, and/or political identity. For example, Palestinians may consider themselves Ramallahan but may be identified as Israeli in the United States; Iranians may call themselves Persian but may be inaccurately identified as Arabs in the United States (Meleis, Lipson & Paul, 1992). The estimated number of Arabs in the United States is 700,000 (Bureau of the Census, 1990).

IMMIGRATION

Most of the original Arab immigrants who arrived in the United States between 1875 and 1948 were Christians from the Syrian province of the Ottoman Empire. They referred to themselves as Syrians, not Arabs. The term *Arab* has come into use only in recent years. Since 1948 the majority of Arab immigrants have been Muslims from independent and frequently rival Arab states (Naff, 1980).

Although there are similarities in all Arabs' traditional culture, variations occur due to separation of communities by water, mountains, and deserts. There appears to be some cohesiveness with respect to language (Arabic, with different dialects), basic religious beliefs, and traditional culture; however, political interests and cultural traits vary considerably. A study of five groups of Middle East immigrants in the United States—Egyptians, Yemenis, Iranians, Armenians, and Arabs—found a number of cultural variations:

• Egyptians spoke a different dialect of Arabic and had their own cultural organizations.

• Yemenis differed from other Arabs in their rural origin. They socialized only with Yemenis and had their own social clubs. Yemenis were significantly less Americanized than Armenians, Egyptians, and Iranians.

• The Arab group identified their countries of origin as Jordan, Iraq, Palestine-Israel, Syria, and Lebanon. They shared a number of social and cultural characteristics that differentiated them from the other four groups in the study.

• Iranians were culturally separate historically, and did not identify themselves with Arabs, although they had some similar cultural characteristics, Islam, and the Arabic alphabet (Meleis, Lipson & Paul, 1992).

COMMUNICATION

Arabic is the mother tongue. Individuals proficient in the Arabic alphabet display remarkable artistic skill using 12 basic design elements in various combinations to construct sentences in a rhythmic geometric pattern (Patai, 1973). Written or "literary" Arabic is used in the modern Arab world in private letters, books, pamphlets, newspapers, public notices, on radio and television news bulletins, and by public speakers. However, few Arabs use this form in everyday conversation. Instead colloquial Arabic is used, and it varies in different parts of the Arab world (Mansfield, 1990).

Iranians speak the Persian language (Farsi), which uses the Arabic alphabet but is quite different from the Arabic spoken by Iraqis, Lebanese, and Jordanians. The Arab ethnic population living near the Iran-Iraq border speak Arabic, and the Kurds of the northwest speak Kurdish (Jalali, 1982). Some Algerians speak Berber (not a written language) as their first language, French as a second, and Arabic only as a third (Mansfield, 1990). Translations of some Arabic expressions are included at the end of this chapter.

SOCIOECONOMIC STATUS

Arab Americans of the early waves (1880–1939) were less educated and spoke less English than later immigrants. Many peddled dry goods; others worked as unskilled laborers in railroad, steel, and auto industries and on farms. Many Arab-American merchants and wholesalers became sponsors for newly arriving immigrants. Thus, the immigrant without funds and knowledge of English, found employment, and the wholesaler found laborers who contributed to the success of his business (Aswad, 1974; Elkholy, 1988).

In sharp contrast, the second immigration wave that started in the 1950s and is still continuing has consisted more of educated elites and technicians. It is estimated that about 78% are Muslims. The family life-style of these professional Arab Americans is fairly similar to that of the typical middle-class white family (Elkholy, 1988).

CHIEF COMPLAINT

Muslims are interested in health care and tend to seek preventive health care to a greater extent than some other immigrant groups (Bullough & Bullough, 1982). In a study of illness complaints (Meleis, Lipson & Paul, 1992) offered by some Middle Eastern immigrants self-identified as Egyptian, Yemeni, Iranian, Armenian, and Arab, the researchers found that Arabs who identified their countries of origin as Jordan, Iraq, Palestine-Israel, Syria, and Lebanon reported more physical symptoms of illness than the other groups. The Arab group showed significantly higher positive morale than both Armenian and Yemeni immigrants. The longer that immigrants had been in the United States, the fewer symptoms or the fewer complaints of illness they reported. Immigration had significant effects on health and illness (Kasl & Berkman, 1983; Hull, 1979).

In another study (Reizian & Meleis, 1987), Arab Americans from Jordan, Egypt, Yemen, Palestine, Lebanon, and Syria reported the highest number of symptoms related to the digestive system (e.g., upset stomach) and the next highest number to the cardiovascular-respiratory systems (e.g., chest pain and difficulty breathing).

Arab Americans perceive themselves as sensitive, with frequent feelings of inadequacy and a potential for being easily hurt by other people's comments. They also describe themselves as being uncomfortable in the presence of authority figures (Reizian & Meleis, 1987).

Weisenberg and Caspi (1989) found that during childbirth, women from the Middle East gave higher ratings of pain and showed more pain behavior than women from Western countries. These findings were especially true for Middle Eastern women of low educational level.

FAMILY

The religious laws of Islam, as interpreted from the Quran (Holy Book), determine family roles. These family laws govern women's way of life and establish males' authority over females with respect to divorce, child custody, marriage, and inheritance (Fernea, 1985). The typical extended Middle Eastern family may cover four to six generations, with lineage composed of all persons who can trace their descent to a common ancestor. The basic structural unit of the family consists of a senior couple, their sons, the sons' wives and children, and any of the senior couple's unmarried daughters. Sometimes other dependent relatives may be included. Traditionally, the family has determined occupations and selected marriage partners for its members.

Traditional Arab Family

The traditional Arab family is based on a patriarchal model; the husband is the senior male and indisputable head of the household. In addition to managing all family finances and properties, he is responsible for satisfying the members' spiritual and material needs. In return, he expects obedience, loyalty, and respect from others in the family (Metz, 1990). In the event of the father's death, the oldest son is responsible for the household, including the care and protection of his mother and unmarried sisters. As parents age, they become more prestigious and are cared for by members of the family.

Intermarriage among close relatives is a common pattern in the Middle East. Relative marriage is preferred particularly with the daughters of the father's brothers or with cousins on the father's side. This practice serves to keep property intact for the patrilineal segment and allows the kin group to maintain an effective social and political position (Elkholy, 1988). In a study of Arabic-speaking individuals in Detroit, Aswad (1974) found that 55% of Arabs interviewed were married to their relatives. Polygamy is sometimes practiced and often justified by the rationale that marriage is preferred over celibacy when there is a shortage of men or that it is better to formalize the male's promiscuous nature within a legal marriage than to force him to have extramarital affairs, as is the case in Western societies (Fernea, 1985).

A father is viewed as prestigious if he has a family with a large number of sons. Traditionally, the position of the family in society reflects on the status of each individual family member. Family solidarity is stressed; each member is obligated to maintain family honor and never to bring shame to the family. Criminal behavior is rare in many Islamic societies (Fernea, 1985).

Some second-generation Arab Americans tend to maintain those aspects of their culture that are compatible with American culture. They usually prepare ethnic foods only on special occasions. Still, many parents enjoy Arabic dishes that their children do not like, so the wife may continue to prepare *mijaddara* or *kebba nayya* for herself and her husband and something else for the children (Elkholy, 1988; Naff, 1980).

Tradition in the Arab-American family life-style was more closely adhered to by the early immigrants than by the more recent professionals. The following list summarizes the major concepts of the traditional family:

• The traditional Arab-American family has been generally patriarchal and usually oriented toward older family members. The elders have been a controlling force in family affairs, including screening and approval of marriage partners for their children, with the father as the final authority.

• Traditionally, a boy has had the right to marry the daughter of his father's brother, and her parents might feel slighted if her cousin did not seek her hand in marriage.

• A woman has been forbidden to marry a non-Muslim unless he converted to Islam before the marriage. If she married a non-Muslim, she and her children would become lost to Islam. However, a man could marry a non-Muslim provided she was either Jewish or Christian, assuming that his wife and children would become Muslims and enter Islam (Elkholy, 1988).

Modern Arab Family

Marriages are seldom arranged today; Christian Arabs and Muslim Arabs usually do not intermarry; and marriage is not encouraged between the two Muslim sects of Sunni and Shia or the two Christian sects of Maronites and Melkites. Marriage frequently takes place between Arab and non-Arab. Arab Christians are more lenient with respect to intermarriages than Muslims (Elkholy, 1988).

Arabs in America are more inclined toward the extended rather than the nuclear family style. The family network serves as a mutual support system in a strange environment (Elkholy, 1988). The need for many Arab-American women to take part in the economic goals of the family has given them a certain amount of freedom from old customs. Many abandoned the veil and long traditional dress after immigration. Third and fourth generations have become somewhat remote from their traditional culture and for the most part are Americanized (Naff, 1980).

Many fourth-generation Arab-American professional families have almost become indistinguishable from other American families of their own class. However, recent immigrants are more nationalistic and seem eager to maintain their traditional patterns. Immigrant leaders are attempting to revive Islamic thought patterns, as well as Arabic language, through classes in the Christian churches and the growing number of Muslim mosques (the term *Arab* includes both Muslims and Christians). Consequently, recent immigrants have successfully stimulated an allegiance and loyalty among many Americanized generations because the tenacious aspects of traditional Arab culture have survived through the efforts of the family and of religious institutions (Naff, 1980).

ELDERLY

Traditionally, the elderly have been controlling forces in the family. Their wisdom has been respected most in families of lower educational levels. As families have become better educated, they have begun to rely more on wisdom gained from science and technology and less on the elders' knowledge based on the past. However, when Arab-American parents retire and are no longer productive economically, they become the responsibility of their American-born children. The elders either live with their children, or if they live alone, their children look in on them frequently.

The Quran gives moral instructions that are an integral part of Islam behavior. Statements such as, "To cherish one's parents is second only to the worship of God" and "Paradise is under the feet of mothers," strongly influence the behavior of Arab Americans in terms of responsibility for the care of their elders (Elkholy, 1988, p. 451). Parents and grandparents are considered an asset and a blessing to the family. Arab Americans are not inclined to consider nursing homes for the care of their elders (Elkholy, 1988).

MATERNITY CUSTOMS AND CHILD REARING

Traditionally, the major events of a woman's life are marriage, pregnancy, and childbirth. In the Middle East the average marriage age for women is 14 to 18, and slightly higher (may be up to 10 or more years) for men. Early marriage for the female might ensure virginity (Fernea, 1985). A woman suspects that she is pregnant when she misses her menstrual period. However, in many traditional early marriages, a woman may not have begun to menstruate before she marries, and later she may become pregnant so often that she rarely sees a menstrual period. Pregnancy is accepted calmly. Activity is not limited during pregnancy, and no special diet is required, but food cravings should be satisfied to prevent markings on the baby (Kendall, 1977). The woman tries to keep her labor a secret from outsiders, believing that their knowledge may adversely affect the labor process (Dorsky, 1986).

Midwives usually assist with the delivery at home. The husband is sent out because of a belief that a man who sees the blood of childbirth may lose sexual interest in his wife. Screaming and loud crying are considered normal during labor; stoicism is neither expected nor practiced. When the birth is about to occur, the woman assumes a kneeling or squatting position assisted by the mid-wife and other close female relatives. Throughout the labor, the mother's skirt covers her legs. When the baby is born, the sex is determined and the nose and mouth are cleared. Then the baby is coated with a special oil and swaddled. (All Muslim boys are circumcised, usually about the seventh day, but sometimes later.) The umbilical cord is cut; and then they await the expulsion of the placenta, after which the mother is helped into bed. Some women believe that the placenta must cool (*abrid*) before being discarded; others believe that it should be washed and buried in some distant place. Neglect of the placenta is believed to have possible disastrous effects on the husband-wife relationship (Dorsky, 1986).

The postpartum woman (*walada*) becomes the recipient of certain privileges and restrictions for 40 days after delivery. She may receive visitors who are relatives and close friends. This treatment is followed even if she has had a stillbirth. It is believed that the *walada* needs special care; she is offered favorite foods and little or no housework is permitted because childbirth is seen as a weakening experience (Dorsky, 1986).

The new mother believes that her infant may be in danger from strangers. She is especially fearful of the evil eye, which is caused by envy and jealousy. Therefore childless mothers are not invited to visit the baby. Statements of admiration for the baby are avoided because they are associated with the evil eye, which can cause illness and even death for the baby (Kendall, 1977).

The infant is cared for solely by the mother after about 10 days. The mother spends a great deal of time looking at her baby, usually without talking to him or her. She carries the infant everywhere she goes and is immensely proud if the baby is a boy. The child is generally breast-fed for about two years. During this time, the mother does not expect to become pregnant; if she does, breast-feeding stops because it is believed that the milk can be harmful to the nursing baby. Supplementary feedings (water-soaked biscuits, soups, tea with sugar) may be started at about 4 to 5 months. By the second year when teeth are in, the child is given adult foods such as rice, yogurt (*mast*), and bread. Consumption of meat by all members of the family is limited. Toilet training is usually begun early, about 8 or 9 months (Kendall, 1977).

Fathers who have had limited interaction with the baby become more involved when the child becomes a toddler. Except for the practice of weaning girls from the breast later than boys, babies of both sexes receive essentially the same treatment. However, by the toddler stage, there is evidence of differences in the treatment and dress of boys and girls. Traditionally males may go bareheaded, while girls are encouraged to wear peaked bonnets until they marry. Boys are given a great deal of freedom and encouraged to be physically aggressive, while girls are kept close to home and encouraged to be sedate and quiet. Misbehavior is readily tolerated for boys but not for girls. Physical punishment is not un-common. Girls are reared in preparation for their future roles of wife and mother. At the age of 4 or 5, a girl may be given some simple household tasks and limited responsibility for the care of a younger sibling. Boys may continue to play (Ghazwi & Nock, 1989).

The Quran and the Sunna (custom associated with the prophet Muhammad) establish that the Muslim child must be protected and cherished; the child, in turn, must be obedient and committed to the will of his or her parents. Sons are expected to obey their fathers even after marriage. The mother's leniency often compensates for the father's stern and dictatorial stance with the children; however, some educated mothers share the stern authority with the father (Ghazwi & Nock, 1989).

A recent study (Ghazwi & Nock, 1989) in Jordan found that compared to Christians, Muslim children tended to retain traditional family behaviors longer. Young Muslims' beliefs and attitudes were found to be quite similar to those of their older generations, whereas younger Christians appeared to be more liberal. Across generations the Christian children displayed greater variation than did the young Muslims.

SOCIALIZATION PATTERNS

Arab Women

The veil (*lithma*) is a piece of brightly colored thin fabric or muslin that is draped around the head in such a fashion as to cover the hair and the forehead. It may be pulled up to cover the entire face except the eyes. This indoor veil is worn by unmarried girls at all times and by married women while doing routine housework or on informal morning visits to friends. The *lithma* is also used when a man unexpectedly enters the gathering place of women. Different types of outdoor veils are worn by women over the age of 10 when they leave the house. The types of outdoor veils and head covers are determined by the women's status and differ by the quality of the fabric used. Women of higher status wear a black outer veil (*sharshaf*), usually of fine fabric and embroidered flowers (Makhlouf, 1979). The traditional practice of veiling is primarily to express modesty, but it can also be provocative and can enhance femininity. Since a veil and long clothing offer a woman anonymity, she can enjoy a certain freedom of movement without being recognized (Makhlouf, 1979).

An Arab woman writer, A'isha Abd al-Rahman, argues that the differing rights and duties of women and men should not imply that women are inferior. It simply means that their roles are complementary. She contends that Muslim women have sufficient latitude to find fulfillment in their lives. She remarks that the Quran shows no gender differences, seeing men and women as equal in the eyes of God. On the other hand, Ghada al Samman, another woman writer who has achieved wide recognition, disagrees with the perpetuation of traditional behaviors. She feels that both Arab men and women need to be freed from constraining traditions, institutions, and beliefs. However, Arab values and customs are still strongly adhered to by at least three-quarters of the non-urban Arab populations in the Middle East (Boullata, 1990).

Arab Concepts

Arab life generally revolves around several extremes—aggression and submission, pride and humility, unity and divisiveness, shame and honor (Patai, 1973). The major values are honor, hospitality, aversion to physical work, courage, individuality, fatalism, and predestination.

It is believed that God predetermines the character and fate of every person and that no one can do anything to alter or influence his or her preordained course of life events. For instance, when a health professional is successful in treating a patient, this success is attributed not to the expertise of the professional but to the will of God. Thus, predestination and fatalism are notable Muslim perspectives (Mansfield, 1990; Patai, 1973).

Similar to other peoples in the Mediterranean, the Arabs use the concepts of shame and honor as bases for their behavior. The acquisition of honor, pride, dignity, and respect, with the avoidance of shame, disgrace, and humiliation, are prime motivators of Arab behavior. Shame and honor define the roles of men and women. For the man, honor is related to fulfilling the masculine role as warrior (if necessary) and fathering children, especially sons. Honor for the woman involves modesty, faithfulness, and the bearing of many children, especially sons (Pryce-Jones, 1989).

RELIGIOUS BELIEFS AND PRACTICES

Islam is a system of religious beliefs that dictates the Muslim (Moslem) way of life. Islam is an inalienable component of Arab culture and is a sociopsychological factor that has stood the test of time. Under Islam there is an obligation of mutual support between an individual and his family and a bond of cooperation for the benefit of the whole between the individual and society (Boullata, 1990). Islam means "submission to the will of Allah" and Moslem means "one who submits" (Chandras, 1977, p. 4).

Muslims believe that God (Allah) revealed the rules governing society to the prophet Muhammad in the seventh century. These are recorded in the Quran, the Muslim holy book. Islam does not distinguish between church and state. Certain behavioral rituals, referred to as the Five Pillars of Islam, must be performed by all Muslims in order to demonstrate and reinforce their faith: (1) a profession of faith by reciting the *shahada* ("There is no God but Allah, and Muhammad is his prophet"), (2) daily prayer (*salat*), (3) almsgiving (*zakat*), (4) fasting (*sawm*), and (5) pilgrimage (*haji*) (Metz, 1990).

The prayer ritual involves praying five times a day: at dawn, midday, midafternoon, sunset, and nightfall. The worshiper prays facing the direction of Mecca using prescribed genuflections and prostrations. Prayers may be performed anywhere, but ideally they are said in a mosque in rows behind a leader (*imam*). Men and women are separated in the mosque, but women generally pray at home (Metz, 1990). The giving of alms, at the rate of one-fiftieth of all income, is an obligation of all Muslims. This money is used for the poor and needy.

Fasting is required during Ramadan, the ninth lunar month, in commemoration of Muhammad's receipt of God's revelations. All Muslims must fast during the daylight hours of the 28 days of Ramadan. Exceptions are made for young children, pregnant and lactating women, soldiers on duty, and travelers on necessary journeys. The month is a time of abstinence from food, drink, tobacco, sexual intercourse, and all other forms of indulgence from dawn until the firing of a cannon at sunset. Each day after sunset there are bountiful family banquets and a night of feasting and celebration. The Ramadan fast is a joyous occasion for Arabs because "it is a time for prayer and self-examination, for sharing good fortune with the poor and disabled, and for visiting family and friends" (Lamb, 1987, p. 100).

The pilgrimage season occurs during the twelfth month of the lunar year when every Muslim (with the means) is obligated to visit the sacred mosque at Mecca (Mansfield, 1990). Muslims who believe that Allah was the true descendant of the prophet Muhammad are called the Shia. The orthodox majority of Muslims are known as the Sunni (Mansfield, 1976, 1990). Ninety percent of Iranians are Muslims who adhere to Shia Islam, whereas the majority of Muslims throughout the world are followers of Sunni Islam (Metz, 1990).

CULTURALLY BASED HEALTH BELIEFS AND PRACTICES

In the context of traditional beliefs, the wearing of amulets containing verses from the Quran is a method of preventing and treating some illnesses. Mothers often obtain Quranic verse from the folk doctor (*mullah*) for their newborn boys to wear in order to protect them from illness. Quranic amulets and coral beads are placed on infants to protect against the evil eye (Dorsky, 1986).

Some traditional women believe that during pregnancy a bizarre creature (*augari*) might grow in the womb of the mother-to-be. The growth of the *augari* is generally caused by emotional upset provoked by the husband. Hydatid mole, spontaneous abortion, any fetal abnormality, and stillbirth are believed to be caused by the presence of an *augari*. If a mother suspects that she is growing an *augari*, she may attempt to destroy it by eating raw onions daily (Dorsky, 1986).

Healers are consulted to protect against the evil eye and mental illness. Healers and pharmacists may be consulted for health emergencies.

CULTURAL DIETARY PATTERNS

Most foods are eaten with the fingers, without utensils. Rice may be rolled in a ball and eaten in this fashion. Whole wheat and plain pita bread are favorites that may be eaten alone, as a sandwich, or with various dips. Sauces are used on most foods. Olive oil is often used for frying foods. Favorite foods include most fresh fruits and vegetables, chickpeas, tomatoes, fried eggs, and teas. Pork and pork products are not eaten by Muslims.

Ethnic dishes include *babaganoush* (eggplant with tahina), *hommous* (chick peas with tahina), *couscous* salad (semolina wheat with raisins and pine nuts), eggplant in tomato sauce with cumin, tabbouleh (cracked wheat, parsley, mint, tomatoes, and peppers), stuffed eggplant (with ground turkey, herbs, and spices), *machshi* (potato stuffed with ground turkey, herbs, and spices), *kubeh* (cracked wheat stuffed with vegetables), *shishlik* (Mediterranean hamburger), and *kabobs* (made with lamb, chicken, or turkey). Frequently enjoyed bakery items are apricot bars, lemon bars, carrot cake, semolina cake, fruit pie, baklava, and halvah.

Muslim food taboos include pork and intoxicating beverages. Except for fish and locusts, animal food is considered lawful only if the animal is slaughtered according to the proper ritual. At the time of slaughter, the person doing the killing must repeat, "In the name of God, God is great" (Ensminger, Ensminger, Kolande & Robson, 1983).

MORBIDITY AND MORTALITY

A survey of 47 Arab Americans indicated that the predominant illnesses experienced in the past year were upper respiratory infections, cardiovascular conditions, hypertension, diabetes, and family and social stress. The health problems reported most frequently were family and marital stress, managing acute illness, adjusting to America, and coping with adolescents (Laffrey, Meleis, Lipson, Solomon & Omidian, 1989).

Some Arabs appear to have a high predisposition to urinary stone disease. Individuals in the Arabian peninsula appear to present a high rate of calcium-containing stones, despite the almost complete absence of hypercalciuria (Mkony, Chuwa, Kahamba, Mteta & Mbembati, 1991; Robertson & Hughes, 1993).

CONCEPTS OF LIFE AND DEATH

Life's goal is to serve Allah and abide by His laws that are recorded in the Quran as revealed to Muhammad. Events in life are predestined. One's socio-economic status is preordained. If one escapes punishment for sins during life, punishment will occur after death. One must confess sins before death in the presence of the family in order to be forgiven. Autopsy is not generally permitted because the body should remain intact (Elkholy, 1988; Mansfield, 1990; Naff, 1980).

Translations of Some Common Arabic Terms

English	Arabic
Nurse	*Mumaridah* (female), *Mumarid* (male)

Doctor	*Tabib* (male), *Tabiba* (female)
Pain	*'Alam*
Out of bed	*Kharig al sarir*
In bed	*Fi'l sarir*
Operating room	*Ghurfal al Amaliat*
Food	*'Akl*
Bedtime	*Wagt el Nowra*
Medicine	*Dawa'*
Treatment	*'Elaj*
Bath	*Hammam*
Family	*'Ayila*

Source: Dag Hammarskjold Library, United Nations, New York.

REFERENCES

Aswad, B. (1974). *Arabic speaking communities in American cities*. New York: Center for Migration Studies of New York and Association of Arab-American Graduates.

Boullata, I. J. (1990). *Trends and issues in contemporary Arab thought*. Albany: State University of New York.

Bullough, B., & Bullough, V. (1982). *Health care for the other Americans*. New York: Appleton-Century-Crofts.

Bureau of the Census. (1990). *Statistical abstract of the United States*. Washington, DC: Government Printing Office.

Chandras, K. V. (1977). *Arab, Armenian, Syrian, Lebanese, East Indian, Pakistani and Bangla Deshi Americans: A study guide and source book*. San Francisco: R&E Research Associates.

Dorsky, S. (1986). *Women of Amran: A Middle Eastern ethnographic study*. Salt Lake City: University of Utah Press.

Elkholy, A. A. (1988). The Arab family. In C. H. Mindel, R. W. Habenstein & W. Roosevelt, Jr. (Eds.), *Ethnic families in America; Patterns and variations* (3d ed.) (pp. 438–55). New York: Elsevier.

Ensminger, A. H., Ensminger, M. E., Kolande, J. E., & Robson, R. K. (1983). Religions and diets. In *Foods and nutrition encyclopedia* (Vol. 2). Clovis, CA: Pegus Press.

Fernea, E. W. (1985). *Women and the family in the Middle East: New voices of change*. Austin: University of Texas Press.

Ghazwi, F., & Nock, S. L. (1989, July). Religion as a mediating force in the effects of modernization on parent-child relations in Jordan. *Middle Eastern Studies, 25*(3), 363–69.

Hull, D. (1979). Migration, adaptation, and illness: A review. *Social Science and Medicine, 13a*, 25–36.

Jalali, B. (1982). Iranian families. In M. McGoldrick, J. Pearce, and J. Giordano (Eds.), *Ethnicity and family therapy* (pp. 289–309). New York: Guilford Press.

Kasl, S. V., & Berkman, L. F. (1983). Health consequences of migration. *Annual Review of Public Health*, *4*, 69–90.

Kendall, K. (1977). Maternal and child nursing in an Iranian village. In M. Leininger (Ed.), *Transcultural nursing care of infants and children* (pp. 19–33). Proceedings from the First National Transcultural Conference. Salt Lake City: University College of Nursing.

Laffrey, S. C., Meleis, A. I., Lipson, J. G., Solomon, M., & Omidian, P. A. (1989). Assessing Arab American health care needs. *Social Science Medicine*, *29*(7), 877–83.

Lamb, D. (1987). *The Arabs: Journey beyond the mirage*. New York: Random House.

Makhlouf, C. (1979). *Changing veils: Women and modernization in North Yemen*. Austin: University of Texas Press.

Mansfield, P. (1976). *The Arab world: A comprehensive history*. New York: Thomas Y. Crowell Company.

Mansfield, P. (1981). *The new Arabians*. Chicago: J. G. Ferguson Publishing Company.

Mansfield, P. (1990). *The Arabs*. Harmondsworth: Penguin Books.

Meleis, A. I., Lipson, J. G., & Paul, S. M. (1992). Ethnicity and health among five Middle Eastern immigrant groups. *Nursing Research*, *41*(2), 98–103.

Metz, H. C. (1990). *Iraq: A country study*. Washington, DC: Federal Research Division, Library of Congress.

Mkony, C. A., Chuwa, L. M., Kahamba, J. F., Mteta, K. A., & Mbembati, N. A. (1991). Urinary stone disease in Dar es Salaam. *East African Medical Journal*, *68*(6), 461–67.

Naff, A. (1980). Arabs. In S. Thernstrom (Ed.), *Harvard encyclopedia of American ethnic groups* (pp. 128–36). Cambridge: Belknap Press of Harvard University Press.

Patai, R. (1973). *The Arab mind*. New York: Charles Scribner's Sons.

Peterson, J. E. (1989, Winter). *The political status of women in the Arab Gulf states*. *Middle East Journal*, *43*(1), 34–50.

Pryce-Jones, D. (1989). *The closed circle: An interpretation of the Arabs*. New York: Harper & Row.

Reizian, A., & Meleis, A. I. (1987). Symptoms reported by Arab-American patients on the Cornell Medical Index (CMI). *Western Journal of Nursing Research*, *9*(3), 368–84.

Robertson, W. G., & Hughes, H. (1993). Importance of mild hyperoxaluria in the pathogenesis of uriolithiasis—new evidence from studies in the Arabian peninsula. *Scanning Microscopy 7*(1), 391–401.

United Nations (1992, March). Telephone interview with an Arab official regarding *Countries of the Arab World*.

Weisenberg, M., & Caspi, Z. (1989). Cultural and educational influences on pain of childbirth. *Journal of Pain Symptom Management*, *4*(1), 13–19.

3

Chinese Americans

The People's Republic of China (PRC) is the third largest country in the world after the Soviet Union and then Canada. The PRC is slightly larger than the United States and is located in eastern Asia, south of the Soviet Union (Summerfield, 1991). Half of the country is covered by mountains, and two-thirds of the area is arid. Ninety percent of the people inhabit slightly more than 15% of the land area.

Southern China is in the monsoon belt, and the climate resembles that of the American gulf states. During late winter and spring, northern China frequently experiences dust storms from the Gobi Desert and the Mongolian plateau.

POPULATION IN THE UNITED STATES

Chinese Americans comprise the largest Asian group in the United States. Numbering about 1.645 million individuals, they represent approximately 0.7% of the American population. Areas with the largest Chinese population are the West Coast and the Northeast. Although Chinese Americans may be found in every state, the smallest Chinese populations reside in the middle states (Char, 1981; Bureau of the Census, 1990). States with the largest percentages of Chinese Americans are California (40%), New York (18%), Hawaii (6.9%), Illinois (3.6%), and Texas (3.3%) (Bureau of the Census, 1988). California and New York have the largest Chinatowns. San Francisco's Chinatown is the original settlement area and the oldest Chinese community in America. Families usually retain their traditional way of life in Chinatowns (Chen, 1980; Spector, 1991).

IMMIGRATION

The early Chinese experienced discriminatory practices in this country because of their skin color and because they were viewed as competitors in the job market since they were willing to work for low wages. Many Chinese immigrants, the majority of them male, took on unpopular work thought to be "women's work" such as cooking and laundering (Char, 1981).

The Exclusion Law of 1882 prohibited the families of Chinese workers from entering the United States, and the Immigration Act of 1924 specifically excluded Chinese women (Kung, 1962; Lee, 1960). Thus, the early Chinatowns in America were essentially bachelor societies, with very few family households. Before the repeal of the Exclusion Act in 1943, the Chinese male-female ratio was six to one (Wong, 1985). After 1943, wives and unmarried children under 20 were allowed to enter as nonquota immigrants, thus facilitating the immigration of Chinese women. After World War II, the War Bride Act of 1945 helped increase the number of Chinese women in the Chinatowns.

COMMUNICATION

The Chinese language has many dialects. The common spoken dialect in China is now known as Putonghua, and its written form is Baihua (Summerfield, 1991). Mandarin is the official Chinese language, but many Chinese in America speak only Cantonese (Rawl, 1992). Other dialects, such as Shanghainese, Mandarin, and Fukienese, may also be heard around American Chinatowns (Wong, 1985). Problems caused by the variety of dialects are overcome by the use of the written language, which is constant (Rawl, 1992). The Chinese language has no alphabet. Words are written as characters using brushstrokes. The system developed to simulate Chinese words using the English alphabet is called the official Chinese Pinyin system. Some common terms are listed at the end of this chapter.

When communicating with another person, Chinese Americans tend to prefer less direct eye contact than Americans and may prefer a side-by-side or right-angle seating arrangement rather than a face-to-face situation. For the most part they prefer not to touch during communication and have been described as a noncontact group (Chang, 1991; Watson, 1970). Some Chinese Americans may hesitate to ask questions for fear of inconveniencing others. Many find it difficult to express strong or negative feelings (Chang, 1991).

SOCIOECONOMIC STATUS

The modern Chinese-American family can be categorized into two groups: the more traditional residents of the Chinatowns, who are mostly blue-collar, dual-worker families, and the white-collar or professional Chinese families, who enjoy a higher socioeconomic status and acculturation level. The latter typically reside in the suburbs, and have integrated into American mainstream society (Wong, 1988). American-born Chinese are generally well educated and usually reside and work not in the ethnic Chinatowns but among the American white middle class. Although not as traditional, many American-born Chinese may retain their values of frugality, respect for authority, hospitality, familism, passivity, and fatalism (Kleinman & Lin, 1981).

CHIEF COMPLAINT

Because many Chinese Americans may be quiet, polite, and unassertive and many tend to suppress feelings such as anxiety, fear, or pain, it is important that the professional health care provider recognize nonverbal signs of discomfort (Chang, 1991). Some Chinese Americans express their emotional distress through physical symptoms (Cheung & Lau, 1982; Kleinman & Lin, 1981). Chinese Americans tend to believe that a good physician should be able to make a diagnosis by the physical examination. Many Chinese physicians make a diagnosis based on the appearance of the client's tongue, which may indicate more than 100 different conditions (Spector, 1991).

FAMILY

Traditional Family

In order to comprehend Chinese behavior patterns, it is essential that we first look at the traditional belief system, the origin of their culture.

Familism is a significant Chinese value. Traditionally, the family has been the major unit of socialization for the Chinese. In the typical Chinese extended family:

- The father, undisputed head of the family, is responsible for the economic support and the discipline of family members.

- The mother is responsible for care of the children and the home. She is subordinate to her husband and insignificant until she gives birth to a son (Lee, 1982).

- Sons are blessings because they carry on the name for the family and ancestors. Boys are so important that in the distant past, girl babies were often killed or given away. Girls were thought to be a bother to feed and care for since they would only leave and marry into another family some day (Char, 1981).

- Filial piety is an important value of the traditional Chinese family system. Sons, and especially the oldest, have specific obligations to the family. They are controlled by their father, whom they call *yeh* ("dignity and sternness") in a patrilocal residence arrangement. Thus, married sons would bring their wives and children to live in their father's house, where the father, the oldest male, would remain the head of the household. After the father's death, the oldest son would become responsible for the household (Char, 1981), and property would be divided among all the sons (Kleinman & Lin, 1981).

Traditionally bloodline relationships have been viewed as more important than marital-sexual relationships; thus, the parent-child bond is often stronger than that between husband and wife. Some husbands are closer to their mothers than to their wives. A wife who does not bear sons is not appreciated, and the husband could divorce her, turn to a concubine, or take in another wife in a polygamous relationship. However, polygamous marriages were generally practiced only by the wealthy (Kleinman & Lin, 1981).

In the traditional atmosphere, the family rather than the individual is the major social entity. The individual exists for the preservation of the family and experiences an identity in terms of the development of the family and its goals. Individualism is discouraged. The family provides a means of communication, interaction, socialization, stabilization, and support (Lee, 1982).

Ancestor worship is an integral aspect of the familism concept. The traditional belief has been that the living and the dead are enmeshed by kinship and descent, and many problems encountered by the living could be avoided by maintaining a balance in relationships with the souls of the dead. Evil spirits or "hungry ghosts" are believed to be souls that were wronged in their lives or were not worshipped appropriately after their death and can cause harm to the living (Kleinman and Lin, 1981). Generally the traditional belief has been that spirits of dead ancestors are always present to protect family members so one must respect these ancestors. Therefore, familism has demanded respect for both the living and the dead (Char, 1981).

Modern Family

A common family type in today's Chinatowns is the nonresidential extended family, which consists of a group of nuclear families, related to each other, who live in separate homes but in close proximity, often on the same street. This grouping may be called a clan. Although these units are independent, they often share a common family business, such as a restaurant or grocery store. In Chinese communities, stores serve as socialization centers for families, other residents, and new immigrants (Wong, 1985).

Many of the first-generation Chinese who arrived in America before 1965, referred to as the "old immigrants," have retained traditional values (the father-son dyad and emphasis on filial piety). The new immigrant families, who arrived in the United States after 1965, are less traditional, tend to prefer the nuclear family model, and prefer that their children affiliate with both cultures, American and Chinese. In China today, many families, especially those of higher socioeconomic status and those who are more Westernized, prefer the nuclear family model. The new immigrants appear to be more affluent and better educated and enter this country possessing more Western values than the old immigrants (Wong, 1985).

ELDERLY

Traditionally, Chinese have treated their elderly with great respect, based not only on recognition of their experience, technical knowledge, and property ownership (in upper socioeconomic levels) but mainly on the Confucian reverence for age. Also, elders were respected because they would soon become ancestors (Morrisey, 1983). However, acculturation may have altered these values, and some modern Chinese youngsters may not show such respect for elders (Chang, 1991).

MATERNITY CUSTOMS AND CHILD REARING

Traditional Practices

Childbirth is a special event for the Chinese family. Traditionally, pregnancy has been the time when the mother has "happiness in her body" (Rose, 1978). Most Chinese mothers prefer natural childbirth, although some may use acupuncture. Some midwives have found it appropriate to allow alternate childbirth positions as preferred by some Chinese women (Sen, 1989). Many Chinese mothers have been described as stoic during labor. When asked about their controlled emotions, some mothers have stated that they would be embarrassed to cry out in front of others. A cultural tendency to control emotions has been observed among the Chinese (Rose, 1978; Chang, 1991).

Traditionally, on the third day after birth, called *kuo-san-jih*, a celebration ceremony is held, and the infant is bathed and dressed in his or her first garments. A special noodle dish is served to the mother, which is believed to stimulate her milk production and hasten her recovery. Food is distributed to neighbors, friends, and all members of the clan. Many families thank the ancestors and pray to them for the health and safety of the newborn. Gifts for the infant create a reciprocal bond between the giver and the baby's family, which is then obligated to return a similar favor at a future date. These obligations have been known to extend through generations (Rose, 1978).

During the first year, the infant is nurtured and kept happy and secure. The child may sleep in the bed with the parents. A permissive attitude pervades during the early years, and the child is not expected to be fully toilet trained until about 4 years of age. In the extended families, grandparents and other family members are available to help with child care (Char, 1981). Children are included in all family activities so that they can learn proper behavior patterns from observing adults. Parents usually refrain from overt praise of their child in an effort to develop humility in the child, but praise is given by nonverbal signs of pleasure, such as a nod or smile. Modern and more Westernized parents tend to compliment their children more often with verbal praise and gifts (Char, 1981).

The traditional father has been the disciplinarian and thus along with the mother has assumed complete responsibility for their child's behavior. First-generation parents are strict disciplinarians, and their authority is rarely questioned by their children. Scoldings and spankings (sometimes with a bamboo rod) are often used as punishment for misbehavior (Char, 1981).

Modern Practices

Modern preferences, beliefs, and practices may be altered in relation to the degree of Westernization and/or acculturation.

SOCIALIZATION PATTERNS

The Chinese have had a traditional philosophy regarding suicide. In premodern China, suicide was not regarded as deviant behavior. Suicide for reasons associated with duty or loyalty were socially acceptable as opposed to suicide committed merely because of unhappiness. For example, a woman who committed suicide after the death of her husband so as not to be forced to remarry and transfer her loyalty was acting in an admirable manner.

Traditionally, the act of suicide was to be rapid and clean, preferably bloodless. Although there were instances of the use of swords and daggers, the most common methods were self-strangulation, poisoning, and drowning (Kleinman & Lin, 1981). Bourne (1973) noted that the suicide rate among early Chinese immigrants was three times the national average. Interpersonal conflicts or a reprimand could provoke a suicide attempt, and this attempt would frequently motivate the family to seek guidance, counseling, and/or psychotherapy (Lee, 1982). Chinese suicide statistics indicate a high female rate as compared to other countries. This rate increases with age. Most common methods of suicide are jumping from a height or hanging. These methods differ greatly from suicide methods used by other cultures (Hau, 1993). The suicide rate of Chinese Americans appears to be lower in states where there is a large Chinese population (Lester, 1992).

Major Chinese personality traits include familism, collective responsibility between kinship members, group solidarity, conformity, and suppression of individuality. Some Chinese have been noted to be strongly past oriented and may experience rigidity of role and status (father-son dyad and filial piety). Chinese culture emphasizes adherence to tradition, loyalty to family, and the relative unimportance of individual feelings. In contrast, American culture emphasizes independence, freedom, and individualism (Rawl, 1992).

Other characteristics observed among Chinese Americans are a desire for harmony and balance, an ability to suppress emotions, stoicism, passivity, frugality, and fatalism. Behavior patterns are often based on a moral code of ethics

(Kleinman & Lin, 1981; Lee, 1982; Wong, 1985). Traditionally Chinese families and schools have stressed moral rules basic to proper behavior, which children are expected to internalize. Kleinman and Lin (1981) noted that the Chinese use moral values as guides to behavior to a greater extent than many other cultures.

RELIGIOUS BELIEFS AND PRACTICES

Traditionally, there have been four major religions of China: Confucianism, Buddhism, Taoism, and ancestor worship. Confucianism was actually not a true religion but more of a moral philosophy. Confucius, born in 551 B.C., developed the first Chinese code of ethics.

Buddhism was developed from the teachings of Guatama Buddha, who lived in India from 563 to 483 B.C. An early form in China was Chan, meaning "meditative." The form of Buddhism that was transmitted to Japan is known as Zen. The underlying principle of Buddhism is that enlightenment is attained through intuitive understanding. Complete absence of thought and nonattachment may be accomplished by sitting and experiencing a meditative state in order to reach the original pure nature of one's inner self (Summerfield, 1991). Buddhism also emphasizes reincarnation, benevolence, self-respect, self-control, and face saving or keeping the family name honorable (Lee, 1986).

Taoism is based on the philosophy of Lao Tzu (or Laotse), who was born about 604 B.C. Taoism emphasizes the mystical aspects of human nature. It professes that immortality is the reward of true faith. Taoism is often associated with health practices. Whereas Confucianism is mainly concerned with the proper way of conducting one's social life, Taoism focuses on attaining the optimal state of well-being for an individual in harmony with cosmological and natural spheres (Kleinman & Lin, 1981). Taoism teaches that life is a cycle, consisting of birth, death and reincarnation (Lee, 1986).

Traditionally, ancestor worship has been based on the belief that the natural and the supernatural are enmeshed in the same world. This religious practice assumes that there is an afterlife and that the living are able to contact the dead (Summerfield, 1991). A shaman (*tang-ki*), or medium, is able to enter into a trance state, where he becomes possessed by supernatural powers and is able to contact dead spirits. Often the shaman is used to seek advice from dead spirits in order to help a believer deal with a problem. By worshiping ancestors, the traditional Chinese family expects to be rewarded by good fortune. Ancestor worship has been practiced in various ceremonies, of which the most important is Ching Ming, or First Feast of the Dead at Spring Festival time (Kleinman & Lin, 1981).

Today, religions practiced in the PRC include Christian religions (Roman Catholic and Protestant denominations) and Islam in the Muslim communities. Many Chinese Americans are affiliated with Christian religions in the United States.

CULTURALLY BASED HEALTH BELIEFS AND PRACTICES

In contrast to the Western health system that emphasizes crisis intervention, Chinese philosophy emphasizes prevention and health maintenance. Many Chinese believe that because the body is a gift from one's parents and/or ancestors, it should be well cared for and properly maintained, and it is best to die with the body intact (Spector, 1991). The Chinese have a holistic concept of health. Psychosocial, physical, religious, and cultural factors are an integral part of the human system. A dominant theme of the traditional Chinese belief pattern is the importance of maintaining harmonious relationships (psychosocial homeostasis) with family and community. Psychological problems are often related to interpersonal stress among family members (Kleinman and Lin, 1981).

The basic concept of Chinese health practices is balance and harmony of energy fields. Since changes are unavoidable in the universe, balance is dynamic rather than static. *Yin* and *yang* are polar terms that describe the contrasting aspects of the universe. Although yin and yang are contradictory, they are also complementary. Their interaction is the essence of all change in the universe. Thus, a yin-yang imbalance within the human body results in dysfunction or disease.

Yin represents the female, negative energy—the passive, unassertive, inhibited, unclear, internal, dark and cold, plus material and concrete human factors. Yin stores the vital strength of life. Winter and spring diseases are yin. Yang signifies male, positive energy—the active, excited, aggressive, external, bright, and hot, as well as abstract and functional human aspects. Yang protects the body from outside forces. Summer and fall diseases are yang.

Body parts correspond to the dualistic concept of yin and yang. The surface of the body is yang; the inside of the body is yin. The front of the body is yin; the back is yang. Body organs are categorized according to yin and yang. Liver, heart, spleen, lungs, and kidneys are yin. The gallbladder, stomach, large and small intestines, bladder, and lymph are yang (Kleinman & Lin, 1981; Spector, 1991; Wollnofer & von Rottauscher, 1972).

Yin-yang dichotomy is also manifested in the polar relationship of hot and cold. Diseases may be classified as hot or cold, and thus remedies similarly classed are used as treatment. Yin conditions are classified as cold, and yang conditions are hot. Foods are also classified as hot or cold.

Yin conditions such as cancer, pregnancy, and postpartum are treated with yang (hot) foods: chicken, beef, eggs, and spicy foods. Yang conditions such as infections, hypertension, and venereal diseases are treated with yin (cold) foods: pork, fish, fresh fruits and vegetables, soy bean curd, and bland foods (Chang, 1991; Chow, 1976; Louie, 1985).

In addition to the cold-hot polarity, other important health theories relating to the body are the concept of breath, the concept of blood, and the concept of wind. Breath *(hay)* is found in the respiratory tract and provides resistance, strength, and freedom from illness. Blood may be weak or strong, and when it does not circulate well, hardened blood vessels and hypertension occur. Lost blood is not regenerated. Wind (*foong*) in the body is noted by bloatedness, passing gas, and foam in sputum (Louie, 1976). *Foong* may be used to describe any disease having an acute (fast like a wind) onset with an unpredictable outcome (Kleinman & Lin, 1981).

Major concepts related to care of the body include balancing, replacement, and moderation. The goal of balancing is to achieve harmony by an awareness of the hot-cold status of the body as well as the status of substances taken into the body. This awareness promotes measures to prevent imbalance, such as eating a balanced diet. Replacement maintains balance. Replacement is the process by which any bodily deficiency can be altered by the use of supplemental foods and herbs. The practice of moderation opposes extremes and thereby avoids the possibility of disrupting the system and throwing the body out of balance (Kleinman & Lee, 1981; Louie, 1976).

For some Chinese Americans, somatization appears to be a common method of expressing emotional distress (Lee, 1982). As a coping method and manipulating strategy, emotions such as depression and anxiety are frequently articulated as somatic rather than psychological distress. For example, instead of regarding depression as a psychological disturbance, the resulting lack of energy and loss of appetite may be viewed as a disturbance in the *chi* (vital energy). Due to sadness, this energy disturbance is detrimental to the lungs; also, too much deliberation is harmful to the stomach and spleen. It is believed that internal organs are centers for both physiological and psychological functions. Thus, the lungs are associated with worries, the gallbladder susceptible to anger and fear, the stomach and spleen affected by thinking too much, and the heart associated with happiness. Emotions themselves are not considered harmful to the body; they are disruptive only when they become excessive (Kleinman & Lee, 1981).

The coexistence of scholarly Chinese medicine and traditional folk healing methods suggests that Chinese Americans will try whatever works. They must use a variety of healing practices: meditation, acupuncture, acumassage, acupressure, marshal arts (kung fu and tai chi chuan), moxibustion, cupping, pinching, and herbology (Lui, 1982).

Meditation is based on the principle of energy systems experienced by the psyche through a trancelike state. It is used to alleviate stress in order to prevent stress-related disease.

Acupuncture is a popular demonstration of the energy fields theory. Fine, hairlike needles are inserted into specific predetermined points in the skin, located on meridians or pathways of energy, *chi*, which lead to various organs of the body. Acumassage, acupressure, and marshal arts (kung fu) use acupoints in the body and the meridians through which energy flows. Western measures, such as the electrocardiogram, electroencephalogram, Kirlian photography, and biofeedback, are similar uses of energy systems (Chow, 1976).

Moxibustion is the application of a heated herb, pulverized wormwood, over specific acupoints of the body. This practice is used to restore energy balance (Spector, 1991).

Cupping is a traditional healing practice in which a heated bamboo cup is placed on selected skin sites. As the cup cools, the skin and energy are drawn into the cup. Pinching, an alternative form of cupping, applies friction to special areas by pinching the skin. These procedures are believed to reduce stress and relieve congestion, headache, and cold symptoms (Chow, 1976).

Herbology is the use of natural elements from plants or animals that help to counteract deficiencies and stimulate the body's *chi*. One of the most popular herbs is ginseng, sold as teas, candies, powders, and tablets in health food stores. Ginseng is frequently used as a rejuvenator. Other uses for ginseng are as a sedative, to stimulate digestion, for faintness after childbirth (Spector, 1991), and to treat hypertension (Change, 1991) and diabetes (Lu, 1986).

The physician has been the primary healer in traditional Chinese medicine. A problem was encountered when male physicians had to treat a woman because men were not permitted to touch women directly. In order to demonstrate areas of discomfort or pain on her body, the female patient used a figurine. Traditionally, women healers were usually midwives or shamans. Female shamans were believed to possess gifts of prophesy (Spector, 1991).

CULTURAL DIETARY PATTERNS

The Chinese American focus on health maintenance and disease prevention is reflected in dietary practices. Food mixtures are prepared with a specific balance in mind. Traditionally, a balance between the foods classed as hot and cold (unrelated to temperature) has been essential to the maintenance of good health. Hot foods (e.g., chicken and beef) are balanced by cold (e.g., fresh fruits and vegetables) (Rose, 1978).

Chinese cuisine is high in vegetables, low in fat and sweets, and high in salt. Vegetables are cooked for short periods to retain the vitamins. Roasts and large portions of meat are not generally eaten. Rather, meat is served in small pieces that can be handled easily with chopsticks. Typical foods include rice, pork, chicken, eggs, various soy preparations, a variety of vegetables, and tea. Milk is not part of the typical Chinese diet because there appears to be an almost universal Asian (94%) intolerance to lactose (Boyle & Andrews, 1989; Char, 1981).

Chinese-American food habits may be summarized by the following:

- Hot and warm beverages are preferred to cold beverages. Hot tea is a favorite.
- Usually raw vegetables and meats are avoided.
- Diets often contain large amounts of soy sauce, which is high in sodium content.
- Diets often include some dried and preserved foods, which are also high in sodium content.
- Spicy foods are sometimes a part of Chinese-American diets (Louie, 1985).

Chinese cuisine is world renowned, and so their foods are enjoyed by many cultures. Notable styles of Chinese cookery are Cantonese, Shanghai, and Sichuan. Cantonese style consists of foods steamed in water rather than fried. Vegetables, prepared to retain their crispness, are combined with a variety of other foods, such as eggs, chopped liver, smoked-cured ham, or prawn slices wrapped in translucent rice flour. Few spices are used, and dishes tend to taste sweet. Shanghai-style foods are somewhat heavier and take longer to prepare than Cantonese cuisine. The longer cooking causes the vegetables to be softer and to absorb more of the sauces. Shanghai style offers more fried foods with more spices. Sichuan uses a liberal amount of spices, hot peppers, and pimientos (Summerfield, 1991).

MORBIDITY AND MORTALITY

Neurasthenia is probably the most frequent diagnosis made by Chinese psychiatrists. Symptoms of neurasthenia include a wide range of complaints: headache, various kinds of pain, pressure and heaviness in the head, noises in the ears, lack of concentration, insomnia, exhaustion, and poor appetite (Kleinman, 1982; Lin, 1983). Kleinman noted that patients diagnosed with neurasthenia most often attributed the symptoms to nonorganic causes, such as work problems, political concerns, family and marital problems, and school crises.

Many Chinese Americans have a lactose intolerance due to a lactase deficiency and are unable to tolerate fresh milk. If this condition exists, the health provider may inform the client about Lactaid and other lactose-free products on the market. Cheese aged over 60 days may be eaten because lactose is converted to lactic acid during the aging process (Chang, 1981).

Chinese Americans manifest a high incidence of the genetic diseases thalassemia and glucose-6-phosphate dehydrogenase deficiency. Thalassemia is a hemoglobin abnormality characterized by a high rate of red blood cell destruction, requiring the client to have frequent blood transfusions. G-6-PD, a blood cell deficiency, causes the production of fragile red blood cells. Individuals with G-6-PD deficiency are prone to anemia in the presence of certain agents such as analgesics (aspirin, phenacetin), sulfonamides, antibacterials (notrofurantoin, choramphenicol, PAS), vitamin K, and quinidine (Molnar, 1983; Overfield, 1985). Another genetic condition found in many Chinese is a marked facial flushing and vasomotor reaction to the ingestion of alcohol, which may explain the low rate of alcoholism among Chinese (Overfield, 1985).

Other observations about Chinese-American health include the following:

- Chinese Americans tend to have fewer dental caries than other Americans (Bullough & Bullough, 1982).
- Chinese Americans have a lower mortality from heart disease (32%) than white Americans (39%) but a higher mortality from cancer (27%) than white Americans (21%).

- Suicide ranks seventh as a cause of death for Chinese Americans as compared to a ranking of tenth for white Americans (Hau, 1993; Yu, 1986).

BELIEFS ABOUT DEATH AND DYING

For the most part, Chinese Americans tend to be stoic and fatalistic when faced with terminal illness and/or death of self or family members. Some Chinese Americans believe in an afterlife, reincarnation, and that the living may be influenced by spirits of the dead, the basis of ancestor worship (Kleinman & Lin, 1981).

Traditional Chinese Americans may abide by *wu-fu*, which categorizes the five kinds of clothing to be worn by mourners to identify the relationship and thereby define the appropriate severity of mourning. This custom emphasizes the family as the basic social unit (Boyle & Andrews, 1989).

PHYSICAL ASSESSMENT

Body Size and Structure

Chinese Americans tend to be shorter at all ages and also tend to complete their growth earlier than most other Americans. They tend to have smaller chest volumes (lower vital capacity) than whites.

Skin and Hair

It is theorized that the yellow color of the Chinese skin is caused by a smaller amount of melanin in the skin than that of African Americans. Also, the coloring may be due to a thickened corium (Molnar, 1983). Chinese-American infants may have mongolian spots, which are irregular areas of blue pigmentation noted primarily in the sacral and gluteal regions of the body. Chinese men generally lack facial hair (Chang, 1991).

Translations of Some Common Chinese Terms

Pinyin is the official Chinese system developed to simulate the sound of the Chinese words using the English alphabet.

English	Chinese
Hello	*noo how*
Thank you	*shiay shiay*
Very good	*hern how*
China	*chong gwoa*
Hospital	*yiyuan*

Nurse	*hushi*
Doctor	*yiesheng*
Family	*jia ting*
Glass of water	*yi bei shui*
Tea	*cha*
Coffee	*fafei*
Toilet	*cesuo*
Today	*jingtian*
Morning	*shangwu*
Afternoon	*xiawu*
Rice	*mifan*
Vital energy	*ch'i*
Hotness	*shu*
Coldness	*han*
Balance, harmony	*t'iao ho*
Blood	*hsueh*

Sources: Kleinman & Lin, 1981; Summerfield, 1991; United Nations, Translations Division, 1991.

REFERENCES

Bourne, P. P. (1973). Suicide among Chinese in San Francisco. *American Journal of Public Health*, *63*(8), 744–50.

Boyle, J. S., & Andrews, M. M. (1989). *Transcultural concepts in nursing care*. Boston: Little, Brown.

Bullough, V. L., & Bullough, B. (1982). *Health care for the other Americans*. New York: Appleton-Century-Crofts.

Bureau of the Census. (1988). *Statistical abstract of the United States*. Washington, DC: Government Printing Office.

Bureau of the Census. (1990). *Statistical abstract of the United States*. Washington, DC: Government Printing Office.

Chang, B. (1981). Asian-American patient care. In G. Henderson & M. Primeaux (Eds.), *Transcultural health care* (pp. 225–78). Reading, MA: Addison-Wesley.

Chang, K. (1991). Chinese Americans. In J. N. Giger & R. E. Davidhizar (Eds.), *Transcultural nursing: Assessment and intervention* (pp. 359–77). St. Louis, MO: C. V. Mosby.

Char, E. L. (1981). The Chinese American. In A. L. Clark (Ed.), *Culture and childrearing* (pp. 140–64). Philadelphia: F. A. Davis Company.

Chen, J. (1980). *The Chinese of America*. San Francisco: Harper & Row.

Cheung, F. M., & Lau, B. (1982). Situational variations of help-seeking behavior among Chinese patients. *Comprehensive Psychiatry*, *23*(3), 252–62.

Chow, E. (1976). Cultural health traditions: Asian perspectives. In M. F. Branch &

P. P. Paxton (Eds.), *Providing safe nursing care for ethnic people of color* (pp. 99–114). New York: Appleton-Century-Crofts.

Hau, K. T. (1993). Suicide in Hong Kong 1971–1990: Age trend, sex ratio, and method of suicide. *Soc-Psychiatry-Psychiatric-Epidemiology, 28*(1), 23–7.

Kleinman, A. K. (1982). Neurasthenia and depression: A study of somatization and culture in China. *Culture and Medical Psychiatry, 6*:177–90.

Kleinman, A., & Lin, T. Y. (1981). *Normal and abnormal behavior in Chinese culture.* Boston: D. Reidel.

Kung, S. W. (1962). *Chinese in American life.* Seattle: University of Washington Press.

Lee, E. (1982). A social systems approach to assessment and treatment for Chinese American families. In M. McGoldrick, J. K. Pearce & J. Giordano (Eds.), *Ethnicity and family therapy* (pp. 527–51). New York: Guilford Press.

Lee, R. (1960). *The Chinese in the United States of America.* Hong Kong: Hong Kong University Press.

Lee, R. N. (1986). The Chinese perception of mental illness in the Canadian mosaic. *Canada's Mental Health, 34*(4), 2–4.

Lester, D. (1992). Suicide among Asian Americans and social deviancy. *Perceptual and Motor Skills, 75*(3 Pt. 2):1134.

Lin, T. Y. (1983). Psychiatry and Chinese culture. *Western Journal of Medicine, 139*: 862–67.

Liu, Y. C. (1984). China: Traditional healing and contemporary medicine. *International Nursing Review, 31*(4), 110–14.

Louie, K. B. (1985). Providing health care to Chinese clients. *TCN 7*(3), 18–25.

Louie, T.T.T. (1976). Explanatory thinking in Chinese Americans. In P. J. Brink (Ed.), *Transcultural nursing: A book of readings* (pp. 240–46). Englewood Cliffs, NJ: Prentice-Hall.

Lu, H. C. (1986). *Chinese system of food cures: Prevention and remedies.* New York: Sterling.

Molnar, S. C. (1983). *Human variation: Races, types and ethnic groups* (2d ed.). Englewood Cliffs, NJ: Prentice-Hall.

Morrisey, S. (1983). Attitudes on aging in China. *Journal of Gerontological Nursing, 9*(11), 589–93.

Overfield, T. (1985). *Biological variations in health and illness.* Reading, MA: Addison-Wesley.

Rawl, S. M. (1992). Perspectives on nursing care of Chinese Americans. *Journal of Holistic Nursing, 10*(1), 6–17.

Rose, P. A. (1978). The Chinese American. In A. L. Clark (Ed.), *Culture, childbearing, health professionals* (pp. 54–63). Philadelphia: F. A. Davis Company.

Sen, D. (1989). Asian culture and communications in midwifery. *Midwife, Health Visitor and Community News, 25*(1 & 2), 16–18.

Spector, R. E. (1991). *Cultural diversity in health and illness.* New York: Appleton-Century-Crofts.

Summerfield, J. (1991). *Fodor's China.* 12th ed. New York: Fodor's Travel Publications.

United Nations. (1991). *Translations of some common Chinese terms.* Unpublished letter. United Nations Translations Division, New York.

Watson, O. M. (1970). *Proxemic behavior: A cross-cultural study.* Hague: Mouton.

Wollnofer, H., & von Rottauscher, A. (1972). *Chinese folk medicine.* Trans. M. Palmedo. New York: American Library.

Wong, B. (1985). Family, kinship, and ethnic identity of the Chinese in New York City, with comparative remarks on the Chinese in Lima, Peru and Manila, Philippines. *Journal of Comparative Family Studies, 16*(2), 231–53.

Wong, M. G. (1988). *A look at intermarriage among the Chinese in the United States in 1980.* Paper presented at the Conference on Racial and Ethnic Relations in the 1990s, Texas A&M University.

Yu, E.S.H. (1986). Health of the Chinese elderly in America. *Research on Aging, 8*(1), 84–109.

4

Cuban Americans

Cuba is the largest island of the Caribbean archipelago, situated in the Atlantic Ocean, between Florida and South America. Because Cuba is located in the tropics, the island experiences year-round warm temperatures and a rainy season that extends from May to October (Rudolph, 1986).

POPULATION IN THE UNITED STATES

Cubans comprise the smallest population of the three major Hispanic groups in the United States (Mexicans are the largest, followed by Puerto Ricans), numbering about 1,043,932 or approximately 0.4% of the American population. This represents an increase of 30% since the 1980 Census (Bureau of the Census, 1990). Within the United States, 70.5% of the Cuban population can be found in the South, 17.6% in the Northeast, 8.5% in the West, and 3.5% in the Midwest (Bureau of the Census, 1992).

IMMIGRATION

The first notable exodus from Cuba occurred when Fidel Castro overthrew the Batista regime in 1959. Many Batista followers immediately escaped to safety in the United States. By 1960, when Castro nationalized all privately owned businesses, the first large-scale exodus from Cuba to the United States began, consisting mainly of middle- and upper-class Cubans who fled to America but had to leave all their savings in Cuba (Bullough & Bullough, 1982).

Quota laws were lenient because these individuals were viewed as political refugees rather than immigrants. (Immigrants are usually individuals in search of economic opportunities; refugees are people escaping intolerable political conditions.) Regardless of motives, the United States officially labeled the Cuban immigration of the 1960s and 1970s as politically motivated, which promoted government programs to assist these exiles (Rogg & Cooney, 1980).

Most Cuban exiles planned to remain in this country only until Castro was overthrown. Eventually they settled down to life in America, many with a determination to make their area of settlement as much like Cuba as possible (Gernand, 1988; Rogg & Cooney, 1980). Most exiles settled where they arrived in Florida. Miami, in Dade County, became the major Cuban center and became known as "Little Havana" (Didion, 1987; Gernand, 1988). About 70% of all persons of Cuban descent in the United States reside in Florida (Boswell & Curtis, 1984). Before the Castro revolution, most Cubans in the United States lived in New York. Union City (West New York, New Jersey) is the second largest area of Cuban settlement. In decreasing order, large Cuban concentrations are also found in New York, Los Angeles, Chicago, Orlando, Fort Lauderdale, Boston, Atlanta, Washington, D.C., Tampa, and Dallas (Boswell & Curtis, 1980; Rogg & Cooney, 1980).

COMMUNICATION

Spanish is the language of Cuba. (See the list of the end of this chapter for translations of some Spanish expressions.) Some Cuban Americans tend to speak rapidly and at a high volume, which may be misunderstood and perceived as a hysterical reaction (Bernal, 1982).

During health teaching or when instructions are given, the health care provider needs to ascertain the client's understanding and approval. Many Hispanics believe that it is rude to disagree or question an authority figure, so they may simply remain silent but not comply (Azziz, 1981).

Generally, individuals of Spanish descent prefer a close personal space zone during personal interactions. Touch is usually acceptable, and a firm handshake is often appreciated by the client and family (Giger & Davidhizar, 1990).

SOCIOECONOMIC STATUS

After arrival in the United States, many of the early Cuban migrants experienced sharp downward occupational mobility. Professionals and white-collar workers had to accept menial jobs, but within a short period many of these migrants, especially the better educated, were able to reestablish themselves in well-paying positions. There are many success stories about industrious Cuban migrants who were able to achieve the good life in America quickly. They became influential in politics, finance, and real estate. As Cuban influence increased, so did their numbers. Miami has become an economically successful city mainly because of the Cuban Americans. Cuban Americans also served as a link between the United States and Latin America and increased business interactions between the countries (Gernand, 1988).

Rogg and Cooney (1980) have noted that better-educated Cuban families were likely to assimilate faster than the poorly educated. They found as well that education and age at arrival facilitated both economic and sociocultural adaptation of Cuban migrants, more so than did length of time in this country. Many Cubans view themselves as middle class and rarely perceive themselves as having much in common with other Hispanics. When Hispanic income was divided into ethnic groups, Cubans demonstrated the highest median incomes, with Mexicans next, and Puerto Ricans with the lowest; however, these data do not reflect the poverty level for some Cubans (Daniels, 1990). Nevertheless, Cubans resist being viewed collectively with other Latins, a behavior that some consider social snobbery (Gernand, 1988).

More than 90% of Cuban migrants to America are considered white. Black Cubans were underrepresented in the early migrations, especially after the Castro revolution, and also underrepresented in the upper socioeconomic classes, who were the major migrants then (Perez, 1980). Some black Cuban Americans reside in the northeast part of Florida and have experienced discrimination in housing and employment opportunities from white Cubans in Miami. The continuing influx of Cubans to Dade County and the continuing segregation practices among white Cuban Americans, black Cuban Americans, African Americans, Jews, and non-Latin whites is believed to be responsible for perpetuating ethnic tensions in the area (Boswell & Curtis, 1984; Daniels, 1990).

CHIEF COMPLAINT

When compared to other cultures (Irish, French Canadian, old American, Italian and Polish) members of Hispanic groups have demonstrated the highest pain intensity and the highest pain expressiveness. They have also been noted to experience the greatest interference with work and social activities and manifest the highest degree of emotional and psychological stress of the other cultures studied (Bates & Edwards, 1992).

FAMILY

The family is the most important social unit for Cubans (Bernal, 1982). Although Cubans are generally found in nuclear families in the United States, they maintain the extended family loyalties practiced in Cuba to individuals who may not live in close proximity. Extended family members who reside in the current household are "family at home." The immediate family generally includes parents, spouse, children, grandparents, siblings, in-laws, and grandchildren. The rest of the family consists of aunts, uncles, and cousins. Close friends, servants, and baby-sitters may be perceived as "just like family" and referred to as "fictive kin" (Pasquali, 1982).

Cuban nuclear families tend to include other relatives besides husband, wife, and children. Often the additional member may be a dependent grandmother who is helpful as a baby-sitter or housekeeper for the family if the mother is employed (Boswell & Curtis, 1984). The cohesive Cuban-American families within their strong ethnic communities serve as dynamic support systems, which decrease the stress of relocation and downward occupational mobility experienced by the new migrants. However, these tight family relationships and strong ethnic affiliations sometimes delay the process of assimilation into American society (Rogg & Cooney, 1980).

Individuals in traditional Cuban families customarily use two surnames. If a man's name is Ricardo Perez Gonzalez, Perez was his father's name and Gonzalez his mother's maiden name. If a woman whose name is Maria Garcia Rivera marries Perez Gonzalez, she becomes Maria Garcia de Perez, dropping her mother's maiden name, retaining her father's name, and adding her new husband's father's name (Boswell & Curtis, 1984).

Traditionally, the Cuban man has been the provider for the family. If he cannot find work, he loses his self-esteem as well as the respect (*respeto*) of his family. Similarly, if a wife must work outside the home, her job also has an impact on the power balance within the family. Sex roles within a marriage have varied among Cuban Americans, depending primarily on socioeconomic factors but also on level of acculturation, time of migration, and religious practices (Bernal, 1982).

Tensions within the Cuban family have stemmed from a greater adaptation of American attitudes by second-generation Cubans, who criticize such traditional practices as chaperoning, and threaten the authority of their parents. Added tensions have also resulted from changes in women's roles. In prerevolutionary Cuba, a woman did not work outside the home since her duty was to maintain the household. Even women with servants in Cuba remained at home to supervise household activities (Rogg & Cooney, 1980). Now, many Cuban-American women are employed outside the home, and in greater proportions than other Hispanic women in the United States (Fitzpatrick & Gurak, 1979).

Today young Cuban-American families are less male dominated, and the roles of husbands and wives are less differentiated than in the traditional family. Unlike many immigrant groups that have undergone a linear acculturation process, Cubans have experienced a three-dimensional process of biculturalism: they have accommodated to the host culture, maintained characteristics of their original culture, and synthesized both Cuban and American characteristics (Szapocznik & Hernandez, 1988).

ELDERLY

Cuban Americans generally prefer to have their elderly cared for by a family member, usually a daughter. The results of a study on caregiving for Alzheimer's patients (Mintzer, Rupert, Lowenstein, Gamez, Millor, Quinteros, Flores, Miller,

Rainerman & Eisdorfer, 1992) found that Cuban-American patients were significantly more likely to be living in their daughter's homes, whereas white non-Hispanic patients usually resided in institutional settings.

CHILD REARING

Traditionally Cubans have believed that for the expectant mother and fetus to maintain a healthy balance with the environment as well as with supernatural forces, the pregnant woman must adhere to a balanced diet, exercise regularly, and avoid envious people and emotional trauma. In addition she should ingest specific teas and herbs, usually recommended by older family members. Any imbalance in the expectant mother's body due to physical, emotional, or supernatural trauma could have serious ill effects on the health and development of the unborn child. In order to protect the fetus, some women maintain the practice of wearing keys on the night of a lunar eclipse, to prevent the child from developing illness or deformities (Dorsey & Jackson, 1976).

Young Cuban children are nurtured and cared for by many members of the extended family. Parents tend to be permissive with their young. Cuban-American children are integrated into family activities at an early age. The mother is the center of family activities, and there is an extremely strong bond between the mother and her children. Many Cuban parents believe that closeness with their children will promote respect, loyalty, and obedience from their children in later years (Pasquali, 1982).

Traditional Cuban families observe *compadrazgo*, in which a set of godparents (*compadres*) are selected for a new baby, before, but, more often, after the birth. The *compadres* offer economic, moral, and emotional assistance to members of the family whenever needed. They automatically become members of the family and must live nearby.

Another important Cuban family tradition is the custom of celebrating a girl's fifteenth birthday by an elaborate and festive party. This *Fiesta de Quince Años* marks the age at which a young lady is marriageable and eligible for increased social activity and dating privileges. In Miami, many *Quinces* are grand and extravagant social events (Boswell & Curtis, 1984; Pasquali, 1982).

SOCIALIZATION PATTERNS

Cuban sex role behavior is based on the idea of *machismo*, which emphasizes masculinity. Adapted from the Spaniards, *machismo* relates to double sex role standards that stress female purity and female marital fidelity but encourage male promiscuity before and during marriage. Traditionally, the term *machismo* has attributed authority and dominance to the male and subservience to the female, compounded by expectations of virginity before marriage and fidelity to her husband thereafter. This philosophy has frequently resulted in marital disharmony within Cuban-American families, especially when applied to working wives and professional women (Bernal, 1982).

Family honor and shame often depend on the appropriate behavior of its female members. Women are viewed as either virgins (Madonnas) or prostitutes. Consequently some Cuban-American parents continue the traditional practice of *chaperonas* for their daughters during dating and courting (Bernal, 1982; Pasquali, 1982).

Choteo—ridiculing or making fun of people and/or situations, exaggerating, and overstating self-criticism—is typical of many Cubans. *Choteo* may also refer to the tendency to downplay the importance of a situation through jokes and satirical gestures (Bernal, 1982; Ortiz, 1974; Rubenstein, 1976).

Another trait noted among some Cubans is referred to as *personalismo*. Cubans are generally friendly and like to minimize personal distance in relationships. In certain situations, they prefer familiarity. Cuban politicians do not like to deal with bureaucratic impersonality, preferring face-to-face contact with a power source. In American politics, *personalismo* is called "power-brokering" (Bernal, 1982; Boswell & Curtis, 1984).

RELIGIOUS BELIEFS AND PRACTICES

Most Cuban Americans are Roman Catholic. Although regular attendance at mass appears to be declining among many Cuban-American Catholics, that does not mean they are not religious. Cubans tend to personalize their religious practices by devotion to favorite saints, whom they view as intimate friends and confidants to worship and seek help and protection in challenging times (Boswell & Curtis, 1984; Gernand, 1988; Rudolph, 1985). The three saints that are frequently most worshipped are Santa Barbara, Our Lady of Charity (the patron saint of Cuba), and Saint Lazarus. Their statues are found in many homes, and replicas in the form of medals are often worn as body ornaments (Boswell & Curtis, 1984).

Santeria, a religious system that blends Roman Catholic principles and African Yoruba tribal beliefs and practices, is practiced by many Cuban Americans (Alonzo & Jeffrey, 1988). Yoruba slaves, brought to the Caribbean during the eighteenth century, associated their deities with Roman Catholic saints (or *santos*); thus *Santeria* means "worship of saints." This folk religion adheres to theological beliefs, magical and medical practices, ceremonial spirit possessions, and exorcisms. It is sometimes perceived as the Cuban version of voodoo. Similar to other Afro-Cuban folk religions, Santeria has an elaborate system of rituals and an acknowledged group of priests, known as *santeros*. Members and other individuals call upon the *santero* to help them interact with supernatural powers, to obtain help in curing a disease, to find a job, and so forth. Although Santeria remains a strong link to the Cuban past, social pressures have caused many Santeria followers to prefer anonymity. Consequently, it is virtually impossible to ascertain the actual number of Cubans who actively or even occasionally practice this folk religion (Boswell & Curtis, 1984; Gernand, 1988).

The diagnosis and treatment of mental illness in some Cuban Americans can be complicated by the Santeria belief in spirit possession (Alonzo & Jeffrey, 1988). In the hospital, it might be appropriate to allow a Cuban-American client to retain a symbolic ornament or medal when going to the operating room or therapy before which jewelry is usually removed. If this item is important to the patient's peace of mind, it should be secured to the client with tape.

CULTURALLY BASED HEALTH BELIEFS AND PRACTICES

Cuban health concepts are based on the principle of equilibrium and balance between the human and the environment (Dorsey & Jackson, 1976). Natural and supernatural forces are inseparable. Good health and well-being are preserved by maintaining a balance between these forces. Mind and body are similarly inseparable; thus illness of the mind can cause symptoms in the body, and vice versa (Azziz, 1981).

The philosophy of balance extends to a cold-hot dichotomy. For example, when related to foods, chile is considered a hot food because it burns the mouth, whereas ice cream and cucumbers are cold foods since they are soothing to the body. During illness, foods that are perceived as appropriate to the condition are consumed. Thus, ice cream and cool liquids are used to treat a fever (Dorsey & Jackson, 1976).

Traditionally illnesses are categorized as physical (organic) or metaphysical. Physical causes have been viewed as a cold-hot imbalance, a deficiency of some essential body substances, or an obstruction. Examples of physical illnesses are *empacho* (obstruction) and *mal aire* (bad air). Obstruction can be caused by excessive ingestion of starchy or heavy foods, which form a ball in the intestines; it is most common in small children. Symptoms of *empacho* are nausea and vomiting, abdominal distension, and diarrhea. These symptoms suggest a diagnosis of gastroenteritis. Bad air may occur when a person with an overheated body (from exercise or fever) rapidly drinks too much cold water or is exposed to a cold wind. Symptoms of *mal aire* are back pain and muscle contraction (*spasmo*), leading to eventual muscle paralysis. Severe respiratory disorders may follow (Azziz, 1981).

Metaphysical illness is due to God's will, magical forces, evil spirits, and/or powerful human forces. Examples of metaphysical illnesses are susto (*fright*) and *mal de ojo* (evil eye). Fright may be brought on by some traumatic terrifying event that causes the individual's spirit to flee from the body. This loss of spirit is indicated by such symptoms as anorexia, loss of weight, listlessness, and pallor. *Mal de ojo* is caused by the powers of a strong person's psyche, intentionally or not, on the physical being of a weaker person. Because of the strong-weak dichotomy associated with this belief, women (especially when pregnant) and children are more susceptible to harm than adult males (Azziz, 1981). A believer in the evil eye concept may perceive a certain illness as resulting from the gaze of an envious person. Some precautions against the evil eye may involve rituals or the use of supernatural forces. Other protective measures are the wearing of a jet multifaceted bead (*una asabache*) or a gold (or jet) charm in the shape of a hand (*un hidago*) (Pasquali, 1984).

The nature of the disease—physical or supernatural—will determine the traditional method of healing selected. If the disease is believed to have a supernatural basis, *santeros* may be the healers of choice. Although there is no clear dividing line between the practices, herbalists may be sought to treat organic conditions (Azziz, 1981). All forms of folk healing have certain commonalities: the client and healer share active roles in the healing process, extensive use of suggestion and hypnosis is essential to the therapy, and the belief that the healer will motivate a cure in a short time is unquestioned. The fact that folk healers activate a therapeutic process within the client's own environment, which allows the client to experience some sense of control, could prove advantageous in the treatment of some conditions (Azziz, 1981).

Santeria practices may be used to treat certain conditions related to illness or other life situations. By 1980, it was noted that over 75 small stores existed throughout Miami that sold Santerian paraphernalia. These stores, called *botanicas*, sell roots, herbs, beads, sprays, candles, incense, potions, and other products for Santeria ceremonies and rituals (Boswell & Curtis, 1984). They also stock the *Orisha*, a book that presents details of certain ritual practices for illness as well as nonillness-related purposes. Many of these items may also be purchased in Cuban *bodegos* (food stores). For nonillness purposes, a few popular potions sold at *botanicas* are *amansaguapos*, said to make a cruel man tender, and *amarrame el hombre*, believed to keep a promiscuous husband faithful (Gernand, 1988).

A coping measure used by some Cuban Americans and other Hispanics is to allude to a number of emotional and psychosomatic complaints. Often symptoms are described in an extremely dramatic manner with various expressions and gestures (Azziz, 1981).

CULTURAL DIETARY PATTERNS

For the most part, Cuban Americans have retained much of their native cuisine because popular foodstuffs are readily available in the Cuban community's supermarkets and grocery stores (*bodegas*). This is particularly true for first- and second-generation Cubans in Miami, New York, and New Jersey (Boswell & Curtis, 1984).

Spain strongly influenced Cuban dietary practices. Cubans adopted the Spanish habit of eating a hearty, leisurely noon meal (*almuerzo*) and a light evening supper (*comida*). Breakfast may be light or hearty, depending on available time. Spanish influence is also attributed to the Cuban preference for spicy, rich foods cooked in oils or wine (Boswell & Curtis, 1984). Cuban dishes are usually hearty, somewhat starchy, and cooked in olive oil, with a liberal amount of garlic and other seasonings.

Pork is the most popular meat in the Cuban diet. Two favorite pork dishes are *lechon asado* (pork roast) and *masas de puerco* (fried pork chunks). Beef is the second most popular meat dish, of which *picadillo* (spicy beef hash) is quite common. Chicken and seafood appear less frequently in the Cuban diet.

Fresh vegetables are not abundant in the Cuban diet, except perhaps for lettuce, raw beets, and green beans, which may be served in salads. Corn and potatoes are frequent ingredients of soups and stews. Beans are a favorite staple in the Cuban diet as a combination of black beans and rice. Two popular bean and rice dishes are *congri* (rice and kidney beans) and *moros y cristianos* (rice and black beans, known as Moors and Christians). Several tropical root crops are also favorites in Cuban cuisine: the yucca, malanga, nama, and boniato (Boswell & Curtis, 1984; Di Perna, 1979). Other Cuban favorites are *cerdo asado con frijoles negras* (roast pork with black beans), *arroz con pollo* (chicken with rice), and *platanos maduros fritos* (fried plantains). Favorite deserts are puddings, pastries, and especially custards (flan; e.g., *natilla* [custard pudding] and *arroz con leche* [rice pudding]). Coffee is the most important beverage. The usually syrupy, dark, bittersweet espresso is known as *cafe cubano*. Coffee with milk (*cafe con leche*) is a popular drink, which is also given to children. Popular alcoholic beverages include Cuban beer (*cerveza*) and rum drinks. The most common are *mojitos* and *daiquiris*, which were invented in Cuba (Boswell & Curtis, 1984; Di Perna, 1979).

MORBIDITY AND MORTALITY

Death Rate

Cuban Americans have the lowest death rate when compared to other Hispanics, as well as non-Hispanic whites and blacks in the United States. Elderly Cuban Americans, including those of disadvantaged socioeconomic status, exhibit relatively low death rates from heart disease and cancer. The homicide rate, although lower than that for other Hispanics, exceeds that for American whites. The suicide rate exceeds that for other Hispanics, whites, and blacks in the United States (Rosenwaike, 1987).

Mortality and Morbidity Rates among Children

Of three Hispanic groups studied (Cubans, Puerto Ricans, Mexicans), Cuban-American women reported the lowest live birthrate (Stroup-Benham & Trevino, 1991), although the infant death rate was lowest among Cuban Americans (Becerra, Hogue, Atrash & Perez, 1991). Of the three Hispanic groups, Cuban-American children have the lowest prevalence of chronic medical conditions, similar to non-Hispanic whites (Mendoza, Ventura, Valdez, Castillo, Saldivar, Baisden & Mortorel, 1991).

Cancer

Cancers of the lung and prostate have been of particular concern to Cubans in Cuba. The death rate for both is lower among Cubans born in the United States than among Cubans in Cuba and whites in the United States. Death rates for cancer of the cervix and rectum among Cubans born in the United States are also low relative to Cubans in Cuba and U.S. whites.

Stomach cancer mortality among Cuban-born men living in America is lower than for men in Cuba and white men in the United States. However, Cuban-born women in the country have higher rates of stomach cancer than American white women. The Cuban-American mortality rates for colon cancer in both sexes and breast cancer in women are intermediate between the lower rates in Cuba and the higher rates among whites in the United States (Shai, 1991).

Diabetes

As compared to other Hispanic groups, the prevalence of diabetes is lowest for Cuban Americans. The relatively low prevalence may be related to socioeconomic, genetic, or environmental factors (Flegal, Ezzati, Harris, Haynes, Juarez, Knowler, Stable & Stern, 1991). However, relative to American whites, the Cuban-American diabetes rate is approximately 50 to 60% higher (Harris, 1991).

Hypertension

Cuban Americans have a higher prevalence of hypertension when compared to the other Hispanic groups. The highest rates are for women, the obese, and those of increasing age (Ford, Harel, Heath, Cooper & Caspersen, 1990).

BELIEFS ABOUT DEATH AND DYING

Because most Cubans are Roman Catholic, beliefs and practices conform to the doctrines of the Catholic church. However, since Santeria is often combined with Catholicism, some may believe in the influence of spirits of the dead as well as Catholic saints. Spiritualists and santeros often attribute causes of illness and death to spirits outside the body (Spector, 1991).

PHYSICAL ASSESSMENT

Cubans range in skin color from white to black. For dark-skinned clients, the skin and mucous membrane assessment techniques described in Chapter 1 for African Americans can be used.

Usually palpation and percussion examination techniques can be used comfortably with Cuban clients, who are generally not adverse to touching.

Thirty-four percent of Cuban-American women are overweight; 8% are severely overweight or obese (Lopez & Masse, 1992). However, of the three Hispanic groups studied, Cuban women appear to display the lowest prevalence of obesity (Nichaman & Garcia, 1991).

Translations of Some Common Spanish Terms

English	Spanish
Yes	*Si*
No	*No*
Doctor	*Doctor*
Nurse	*Enfermera*
Thank you	*Gracias*
Family	*Familia*
Clergy	*Clero*
Pain	*Dolor*
Itch	*Picor*
Hot	*Caliente*
Cold	*Frio*
Weak	*Cansado*
Short of breath	*Falta de respiracion*
Allergic	*Alergia*
Need to go to bathroom	*Ir al bano*
Need bedpan	*Chata*
Need bed raised	*Cama/aumento*
Need bed lowered	*Cama/baja*
Need a blanket	*Frisa*
Need pills	*Pilduras*
Water	*Agua*
Milk	*Leche*
Juice	*Jugo*
Glasses	*Espejuelos*
Leave me alone	*Dejeme solo*
Get out of bed	*Levantarme*
Back to bed	*A cama*
Open door	*Puerta abierta*

| Close door | *Puerta cerrada* |
| Change | *Cambielo* |

Source: Beamatic Communicator. Courtesy of Omnimed Inc., Pine Avenue, P.O. Box 446, Maple Shade, NJ 08052–0446.

REFERENCES

Alonzo, L., & Jeffrey, W. D. (1988). Mental illness complicated by the Santeria belief in spirit possession. *Hospital Community Psychiatry*, *39*(11), 1188–91.

Azziz, R. (1981, July). The Hispanic patient. *Pennsylvania Medicine*, 22–25.

Bates, M. S., & Edwards, W. T. (1992). Ethnic variations in the chronic pain experience. *Ethnicity and Disease*, *2*, 63–83.

Becerra, J. E., Hogue, C. J., Atrash, H. K., & Perez, N. (1991). Infant mortality among Hispanics: A portrait of heterogeneity. *Journal of the American Medical Association*, *265*(2), 217–21.

Bernal, G. (1982). Cuban families. In M. McGoldrick, J. K. Pearce & J. Giordano (Eds.), *Ethnicity and family therapy* (pp. 187–207). New York: Guilford Press.

Boswell, T. D., & Curtis, J. R. (1984). *The Cuban-American experience: Culture, images and perspectives*. Totowa, NJ: Rowman & Allanheld Publishers.

Bullough, V. L., & Bullough, B. (1982). *Health care for the other Americans*. New York: Appleton-Century-Crofts.

Bureau of the Census. (1992). *Statistical abstract of the United States*. Washington, DC: Government Printing Office.

Daniels, R. (1990). *Coming to America: A history of immigration and ethnicity in American life*. New York: Harper Collins.

Didion, J. (1987). *Miami*. New York: Simon and Schuster.

Di Perna, P. (1979). *The complete travel guide to Cuba*. New York: St. Martin's Press.

Dorsey, P. R., & Jackson, H. Q. (1976). Cultural health traditions: The Latino/Chicano perspective. In M. F. Branch & P. P. Paxton (Eds.), *Providing safe nursing care for ethnic people of color* (pp. 41–80). New York: Appleton-Century-Crofts.

Fitzpatrick, J., & Gurak, D. T. (1979). *Hispanic intermarriage in New York City*. New York: Hispanic Research Center, Fordham University.

Flegal, K. M., Ezzati, T. M., Harris, M. I., Haynes, S. G., Juarez, R. Z., Knowler, W. C., Perez-Stable, E. J., & Stern, M. P. (1991). Prevalence of diabetes in Mexican Americans, Cubans, and Puerto Ricans from Hispanic Health and Nutrition Examination Survey, 1982–1984. *Diabetes Care*, *14*(7), 628–38.

Ford, E. S., Harel, Y., Heath, G., Cooper, R. S., & Caspersen, C. J. (1990). *Journal of Clinical Epidemiology*, *43*(2), 159–65.

Gernand, R. (1988). *The Cuban experience: The people of North America*. New York: Chelsea House Publishers.

Giger, J. N., & Davidhizar, R. (1990). Transcultural nursing assessment: A method for advancing nursing practice. *International Nursing Review*, *37*(1), 199–201.

Harris, M. I. (1991). Epidemiological correlates of NIDDM in Hispanics, whites, and blacks in the U.S. population. *Diabetes Care*, *14*(7), 639–48.

Lopez, L. M., & Masse, B. (1992). Comparison of body mass indexes and cutoff points for estimating the prevalence of overweight in Hispanic women. *Journal of the American Diabetic Association, 92*(11), 1343–47.

Mendoza, F. S., Ventura, S. J., Valdez, R. B., Castillo, R. O., Saldivar, L. E., Baisden, K., & Martorell, R. (1991). Selected measures of health status for Mexican Americans, mainland Puerto Rican, and Cuban American children. *JAMA, 265*(2), 227–32.

Mintzer, J. E., Rupert, M. P., Lowenstein, D., Gamez, E., Millor, A., Quinteros, R., Flores, L., Miller, M., Rainerman, A., & Eisdorfer, C. (1992). Daughters' caregiving for Hispanic and non-Hispanic Alzheimer patients: Does ethnicity make a difference? *Community Mental Health Journal, 28*(4), 293–303.

Nichaman, M. Z., & Garcia, G. (1991). Obesity in Hispanic Americans. *Diabetes Care, 14*(7), 691–94.

Ortiz, F. (1974). *Neuvo Catauro de Cabanismos*. Havana: Editorial de Ciencias Sociales.

Pasquali, E. A. (1982). *Assimilation and acculturation of Cubans on Long Island*. Unpublished doctoral dissertation, State University of New York at Stony Brook, New York.

Pasquali, E. A. (1984, May–June). The evil eye phenomenon; Its implications to community health nursing. *Home Healthcare Nurse*, pp. 32–35.

Perez, L. (1980). Cubans. In S. Thernstrom (Ed.), *Harvard encyclopedia of American ethnic groups* (pp. 256–60). Cambridge: Belknap Press of Harvard University Press.

Rogg, E. M., & Cooney, R. S. (1980). *Adaptation and adjustment of Cubans: West New York, New Jersey, Bronx*. New York: Hispanic Research Center, Fordham University.

Rosenwaike, I. (1987). Mortality differentials among persons born in Cuba, Mexico, and Puerto Rico residing in the United States. *American Journal of Public Health, 77*(5), 603–6.

Rubenstein, D. (1976). Beyond the cultural barriers: Observations of emotional disorders among Cuban immigrants. *International Journal of Mental Health, 5*(2), 69–79.

Rudolph, J. D. (1985). *Cuba: A country study*. Washington, DC: American University, Foreign Areas Studies.

Shai, D. (1991). The cancer mortality in Cuba and among the Cuban-born in the United States, 1979–1981. *Public Health Report, 106*(1), 68–73.

Spector, R. E. (1991). *Cultural diversity in health and illness* (3d ed.). Norwalk, CT: Appleton & Lange.

Stroup-Benham, C. A., & Trevino, F. M. (1991). Reproductive characteristics of Mexican-American, mainland Puerto Rican, and Cuban-American women: Data from the Hispanic Health and Nutrition Examination Survey. *Journal of the American Medical Association, 265*(2), 222–26.

Szapocznik, J., & Hernandez, R. (1988). The Cuban American family. In C. H. Mindel, R. W. Haberstein & R. Wright, Jr. (Eds.), *Ethnic families in America: Patterns and variations* (3d ed.) (pp. 160–72). New York: Elsevier.

Wald, K. (1978). *Children of Che: Childcare and education in Cuba*. Palo Alto, CA: Ramparts Press.

Zimbalist, A. (1987). *Cuba's socialist economy toward the 1990s*. Boulder, CO: Lynne Rienner Publishers.

5

East Indian Americans

The Republic of India, often referred to as the Indian subcontinent, is commonly called India. Twenty-five states plus seven centrally administered union territories comprise the Indian subcontinent (Government Publication of India, 1993; Kamar, 1994). India is located in Asia, southeast of the People's Republic of China (PRC). The country is surrounded by the Bay of Bengal in the east, the Arabian Sea in the west, and the Indian Ocean on the south. To the north, India shares land boundaries with Pakistan, Nepal, the PRC, Bangladesh, Burma, and Bhutan. Mount Everest and the Himalayas, the highest mountains in the world, extend along India's northern boundary (Government Publication of India, 1993; Nyrop, 1986).

The Himalayan range to the north acts as a meterorological barrier so that the monsoon rhythm is apparent throughout most of the country. Although the major portion of northern India lies beyond the tropical zone, generally the country has a tropical climate marked by relatively high temperature and dry winters. However, temperature variation may be noted, from the subfreezing temperatures of the snow-covered Himalayan ranges to the year-round tropical weather of the southern peninsula (Government Publication of India, 1993; Nyrop, 1986).

Despite its immense size, India is overpopulated. It is a heterogeneous subcontinent with respect to physical, economic, religious, racial, social, and cultural variations (Wasan, 1990). India has a large and diverse mixture of races, with all of the five major racial types represented: Australoid, Mongoloid, Europoid, Caucasian, and Negroid (Government Publication of India, 1993).

Throughout its modernization, India has preserved its ancient civilization and has never lost sight of the ideals that gave it strength through the centuries. Its composite culture has made it a truly vibrant democracy. Science and technology have provided the tools for improving the lot of its poor, but this nation of over 900 million continues to live with some of its traditions that date back 4,000 years or more (Government Publication of India, 1993).

POPULATION IN THE UNITED STATES

East Indian Americans number approximately 815,000 individuals, representing 0.3% of the American population. East Indians or Asian Indians are the fourth largest Asian group in the United States. Asian groups in decreasing number order are Chinese, Filipinos, Japanese, Asian Indians, Koreans, and Vietnamese (Bureau of the Census, 1992).

The largest number of East Indian Americans live in San Francisco and Los Angeles. Other large concentrations are found in New York City, especially Flushing and Queens, as well as in Jersey City and Westchester and Washington, D.C. Major East Indian communities exist in Illinois, Pennsylvania, Ohio, Michigan, Massachusetts, Maryland, and Texas. Approximately 85% of these individuals are Caucasian (Jensen, 1980).

IMMIGRATION

The East Indian Americans in the United States and their descendents, who frequently refer to themselves as Asian Indians or Indo-Americans, are from both southern and northern India (Kamar, 1994). The largest group migrated to America after 1965 when immigration law eliminated national quotas.

COMMUNICATION

India has about 15 major languages and 844 dialects. The Sanskrit of the Aryan settlers merged with the earlier Dravidian vernaculars and gave rise to new languages. Hindi, spoken by 45% of the population, is the national language. English is the language used for official communication (Government Publication of India, 1993). One embassy official stated that altogether there may be 18 languages (a number that includes English as well as 2 recently added languages) spoken in India (Kamar, 1994). Besides Hindi, the most commonly used of the languages are Bengali, Punjabi, Gujarati, and Urdu of the Indo-Aryan linguistic family and Tamil of the Dravidian family (Jensen, 1980). Individuals in public life and those of higher socioeconomic status most frequently speak Hindi and English (Kamar, 1994; Nyrop, 1986).

East Indian Americans are polite and courteous and highly respectful of authority figures. Women may show more distance with male superiors than with female counterparts. Many East Indian Americans practice the traditional greeting, head bowed and hands clasped in prayer fashion while the individual says *namaste*, the Hindi word for (''I bow to you'') (Miller & Supersad, 1991; Patibandla, 1994).

When the East Indian–American client is a woman accompanied by an older woman or her husband, the health professional should remember to greet the husband or the older person first. During the health history, the female client may allow her husband or elder to give most of the information. A woman generally will not maintain eye contact with a male health professional, especially in her husband's presence (Miller & Supersad, 1991).

Many East Indian Americans display a soft-spoken manner with frequent head and hand movements to add vitality to their words. Men usually maintain direct eye contact with each other when conversing, but some women may look down when addressing their husbands and older male relatives as a sign of respect. Affectionate touching and public shows of affection with family and friends are not socially acceptable behaviors among many East Indian Americans (Miller & Supersad, 1991). Many of these characteristic behaviors are no longer observed among the younger, modern East Indian Americans.

SOCIOECONOMIC STATUS

Socioeconomic status is related to the caste system, a traditional religious-cultural method of structuring life. The system establishes and maintains highly defined social levels that permeate all religious, linguistic, and ethnic associations. This traditional system is practiced in some of the Indian villages; however, many of these practices have changed with population shifts to the cities of India and migration to the United States.

Traditional beliefs held that purity was essential to one's interaction with the gods. Brahman priests, the highest rank, were the purest. In contrast, the untouchables, the lowest order, performed the most polluting duties (those that placed them in contact with pollutants such as human excrement, human hair and nails, water, garbage, and corpses) (Nyrob, 1986). Intermediate castes were: second to the Brahman, the Kshatriya (warriors); the Vaisya (farmers and merchants); and finally, just above the untouchables, the Sudras (poor farmers and artisans). Mahatma Gandhi named the untouchables *Harijans* (people of God) (Fishlock, 1983). Traditionally, many believed that the only emancipation from a particular caste or level in society was to be reborn into a higher caste (Miller & Supersad, 1991).

The Brahmans, the most prestigious, tended to be lighter in color; the Sudras, who performed menial tasks for the higher groups, tended to be darker skinned. After the Aryans from Central Asia invaded India, the original inhabitants fled to the south and were called Dravidians. The Aryans tend to be fair, whereas the Dravidians tend to be dark skinned (Patibandla, 1994). In the north where the climate is colder, the inhabitants tend to be fairer; in the south where the climate is tropical, the inhabitants tend to be darker complexioned (Kamar, 1994; Miller & Supersad, 1991).

A typical village in India may consist of several castes or social levels. Each caste level is called a *jati*, and broader and more general divisions within the caste system are called *varnas*. However, *jati* (of which there are approximately 3,000 in contemporary society), rather than *varnas*, tend to be the functional categories of the Indian caste system (Nyrop, 1986).

The traditional caste structure has been related to kinship, with all of a person's kin belonging to the same *jati*. Caste affiliation is patrilineal, so children are members of their father's *jati*. Traditionally, marriage was arranged by kin, and partners were selected from among *jati* mates, ensuring the perpetuation of the caste system. Also, the *jati* influenced the availability of health and social services and scholarships for education. Traditionally, *jati* affiliation may have determined an individual's occupation. Nepotism often enhanced an individual's employment and business opportunities (Aris, 1990; Nyrop, 1986). Because a village may contain anywhere from 2 to 30 different *jati*, the *jati* system provided an interdependent service network by which occupational specialization integrated the various *jatis* in a symbiotic relationship. However, since *jatis* in the cities were frequently a source of economic competition, caste system practices were modified in major urban areas (Nyrop, 1986).

CHIEF COMPLAINT

Hindus tend to be stoic and seldom complain about illness or pray for health. They may not readily discuss their chief concern or complaint, past illness or family history required for the health assessment. Many Hindus believe that self-control of feelings is one of the keys to maintaining the wellness state.

FAMILY

Family Structure

Traditionally, the family structure of India has been patriarchal and patrilineal, and the residential norm is patrilocal. The preferred joint household consisted of a senior couple, their unmarried children, their married sons' families, and perhaps the parents of the senior couple (particularly the husband's mother) and any other relatives (Nyrop, 1986). A major function of the family was to ensure its continuity through the production of male heirs. All family property was divided evenly among the males, regardless of age. The female portion consisted only of the amount that would be given to the daughter's husband as a dowry when she married (Nyrop, 1986). An important traditional family value was concern for the welfare of the family as a whole. Individual members were expected to make sacrifices and pool their resources for the benefit of the total family unit (Chekki, 1988).

Traditional Marriage and Spousal Roles

The Musali villagers in South India believed in a religious ideology known as Pativratya, which has governed the lives of Hindu women. Pativratya ideology, based on an androcentric (male worship) theory, holds that males are physically strong, pure, and emotionally mature. Women maintained purity of body through virginity before marriage and chastity after. The man's responsibility is to maintain this pure state, even if it infringes on the woman's freedom, for only through a state of purity can a woman give birth to the children a man must have to perpetuate his family. Marriages were generally arranged by the families, often without the consent of the bride and groom (Dhruvarajan, 1988). A Pativratya woman was taught that her life's goal was to be of service to her husband. She existed solely for the comfort of her husband (her lord and master). Thus, she ate and slept only after he was satisfied and made comfortable. She never sat when he was standing. To demonstrate his authority and her subordination, she always walked behind him. The marital union was thus not a companionship relationship but an authority relationship (Dhruvarajan, 1988).

Chekki (1988) studied a Lingayat community and found a somewhat different philosophy. The Lingayat religion professed that there is no life after death, so one must strive toward unity with God through purity and proper actions in the present life. Lingayat women enjoyed equality with men, and thus their ideology of egalitarianism opposed the traditional Hindu system of inequality and subordination of women. Lingayat ideology encompassed concepts of community sharing, thrift, sobriety, modernization, and nonviolence. Family values focused on the importance of the total unit above the interests of the individual (Chekki, 1988).

Traditional Lingayat marriages were also arranged. Approximately 40% were marriages among kin (consanguineous unions). The custom of dowry prevailed, and the divisions of labor within the family were gender role related. Although the husband-wife relationship was not based on love at marriage, it was expected that they would eventually develop a love relationship after continued intimacy. The father was the authoritarian figure of the family; the mother was the central figure through her love, affection, and nurturing functions. A high achievement motivation was typical of Lingayat families (Chekki, 1988).

Traditionally, marriage was the normal and most respectable state for Indians, important to both the marriage partners and to maintain the respectable status of the family and *jati*, as well as to unite two families (Nyrop, 1986). Unmarried daughters past the age of 25 were a poor reflection on the family. In traditional India, divorce was not common. Divorce today in India poses no problem for a man, but in some areas, it could lower the social status of a woman unless she is wealthy and/or well educated (Patibandla, 1994).

Marriage arrangements differ somewhat in southern and northern India. Although consanguineous marriages are frequently found in the southern regions, today they tend to be with less close kin. Some castes prefer marriage between a man and the daughter of his eldest sister (that is, a mature uncle and his young niece). The marriage between a woman and her mother's brother (again, young niece and older uncle) is also an acceptable union. Typically, the next preference is marriage between first cousins. The age gradient is always important. The bride's age usually ranges from 16 to 21 (frequently about 18), and the groom is in his late twenties or older. Depending on the caste community, the frequency of kin marriage still exists in several regions of South India (Driver & Driver, 1988; Patibandla, 1994).

Some nonsanguineous marriages are arranged through advertisements in the matrimonial columns of Indian newspapers. Also, communities in the United States advertise in Indian association papers here, including *Hindu*, *India Abroad*, and the Indian Cultural Association papers. Another source of communication and advertisement is through *India Digest*, a cultural interest group connected throughout the world by a computer network (Rajamani, 1994). Advertisers seek a match that is suitable in terms of desirable caste, language, and age. Marriage to a permanent resident of the United States or Canada, or someone with a green card, could be advantageous to a partner wishing to migrate. Matrimonial agencies charge a relatively high fee for arranging migration marriages (Bhargava, 1988; Nyrop, 1986).

CHILD REARING

East Indian American mothers are devoted and nurturing to their children. Mothers are expected to make sacrifices for their families and are highly respected. Traditionally in India, the cow has been sacred because it is a symbol of motherhood (Sarin, 1985).

Traditionally, the birth of a child is a happy occasion, and many relatives and friends are expected to visit the family and new baby. A special ceremony, the *Naamkaran*, is held to name the baby. Several other religious ceremonies are devoted to children. During the ceremony of *Mundan*, Hindu boys have their heads shaved, because it is believed that keeping original hair from birth causes bad luck. Sikh boys do not cut their hair but are given their first *puggree* (turban) at a ceremony, *Dastar Bandi*. Muslim children are introduced to their holy book, the Quran, in the *Bismillah* ceremony, and before they are 13, they are taught how to fast for the month of Ramzan in the ceremony of *Roza Rakha* (Sarin, 1985). Brothers and sisters have a close emotional bond, celebrated annually in the festival of *Raksha Bandhan*, when the sister places a bracelet (*rakhi*) on her brother's wrist as a symbol of love and loyalty to each other (Sarin, 1985).

The emotional bond between mother and daughter is usually strong. Traditionally, after the age of 10, a daughter is kept close to her mother, to be carefully taught and prepared for her future life as a wife and mother. She is taught how to cope with a difficult husband and/or a demanding mother-in-law, how to lower herself and show deference, and how to suffer silently. The mother serves as a role model for her daughter, who will later be judged by her mother's behavior. When considering the daughter as a marriage partner, the prospective groom's family places great importance on the belief, "like mother, like daughter" (Dhruvarajan, 1988).

Tradition has it that a son is allowed much freedom and socializes freely. The teenage boy may begin to associate with his father at times. The eldest son, who continues the family name and will be responsible for performing the holy death rites at the father's funeral, is usually the closest to the father (Miller & Supersad, 1991).

Although the mother is close to her daughter, there may be a stronger bond with her son, who will take care of her in her old age while her daughters live with their in-laws. Mothers may compromise the interests of their daughters for those of their sons. The close bond between mother and son can cause problems when the son's wife enters the home and the mother has to share her son with another woman. Therefore, fear of mistreatment by the mother-in-law has always been a major concern of young brides. A few reports exist of disastrous mishaps befalling young brides who could not get along with their mother-in-law (Dhruvarajan, 1988; Nyrop, 1985; Patibandla, 1994).

East Indian parents place high value on education for their children. In India the level of literacy is 52% (Patibandla, 1993). East Indian Americans have a higher rate of college graduates than the average American population and thus enjoy a relatively lower poverty rate than the rest of the population in the United States (Miller & Supersad, 1991).

Operation Blackboard was launched in India in 1990 to achieve universalization of primary education. In many areas of India, government education policy reflects a special concern for girls. India received international recognition for commitment to the achievement of Education for All (EFA) at the world conference on EFA in March 1990 (Government Publication of India, 1993).

ELDERLY

Traditionally the Indian mother-in-law or grandmother and eldest son are frequently the most important family decision makers. The mother-in-law is often the main decision maker in family health care practices (Kakar, Chopra, Samuel & Sangar, 1989; Miller & Supersad, 1991).

SOCIALIZATION PATTERNS

Some East Indian American family systems may encourage timidity, laissez-faire, dependency, humility, and deference in their members. Women tend to be stoic and self-sacrificing (Miller & Supersad, 1991). The East Indian–American way of life, especially that of tolerance, accommodation, and docility, has facilitated their assimilation into American society. In addition most adhere to the middle-class value system in America (Chandras, 1977).

Many East Indian–American women wear the traditional long, gracefully draped sari. Others may wear soft pants (*salwar*) with a long top (*kameez*) and scarf (*dupatta*) (Ratnaraj, 1994). A fashionable married woman may wear a dot on her forehead, colored to coordinate with her outfit. Earrings in the ears and/or an earring in the side of the nose are also decorative and fashionable. East Indian men generally wear Western attire. However, attire is generally determined by the area of India where the person resides. Sikh men usually wear turbans in public (Indian Consulate General Information Section, 1991).

RELIGIOUS BELIEFS AND PRACTICES

Hinduism, probably the oldest religion in the world, is practiced by 80% of the people of India. The Hindu religion has its origin in the concepts of the early Aryans who came to India more than 4,000 years ago. Hinduism is not merely a religion but also a philosophy and way of life. It teaches the immortality of the human soul and the ultimate union of the individual with the all-pervasive spirit. The self is eternal, changeless, and ancient and is never destroyed, even when the body is destroyed. Hinduism respects other religions and does not seek converts (Government Publication of India, 1993).

The practice of Hinduism varies depending on geography, socioeconomic status, family custom, and personal preference. Hindu individuals may be monotheistic or polytheistic, or even atheistic. The formal house of worship is the temple. Many worship regularly at home and at the temples during festivals. Hinduism's theological rationale is based on a body of sacred literature known as the Vedas, which was composed between 1200 and 600 B.C. (Nyrop, 1986).

To the Hindu believer, religion is a spiritual expression of the reality of the universe. The knowledge of reality is the ultimate goal. Only specially gifted individuals can achieve a state of high spiritualism, enabling them to know the truth. They are then said to experience *Moksha* (or *mukti*), which means "release from the false illusions of the external world." This heightened state of spiritualism may be reached through exercise of the intellect, devotion to deities, expansion of the senses, heightened control of the body, and disciplined meditation.

It is believed that the divine spirit permeates the universe, and people perceive the divine in accordance with their spiritual level. All life forms (including animals and gods) exist as a hierarchy, depending on spiritual advancement or purity. Many life forms pass through a chain of incarnations, thus assuming various positions in a hierarchy during their different lives. All souls are considered equal; thus, the rationale for the principle of *ahimsa* (noninjury to living things) is manifested in the practice of vegetarianism (Nyrop, 1986).

The law of karma determines life cycles through birth and rebirth. Karma is the spiritual merit or demerit that an individual acquires during his or her lives. Thus, all lives are ordered in a hierarchy dependent on one's moral behavior in a previous life. Perfection of karma leads to emancipation from the burdens of birth and rebirth. (In Buddhism, this release is known as nirvana.)

Reincarnation is the central belief of Hinduism. The Hindu's goal in life is to acquire the highest spiritual merit or karma that will determine his or her future lives. Each Hindu strives for a final release from the burden of birth and rebirth, which can be achieved only through a knowledge of truth and the experience of reality. Reality will be understood when there is a spiritual union of the individual soul and the universal soul. This ultimately desirable state may be attained by only a few of the purest and most highly spiritual, who are thereby released from the burden of reincarnation (Boyle & Andrews, 1989; Nyrop, 1986).

Among the other religions practiced by East Indians are Buddhism, Jainism, Islam, Sikhism, Zoroastrianism, Christianity, and Judaism (Government Publication of India, 1993; Nyrop, 1986). The majority of East Indian Americans are Hindus. Although Sikhs represent only 2% of the population in India, Sikhs are about 30 to 40% of the East Indian population in California. Muslims, Jains, and Zoroastrians make up small groups in both the homeland and America (Jensen, 1990).

CULTURALLY BASED HEALTH BELIEFS AND PRACTICES

East Indians generally believe that health is based on the body's intrinsic ability to heal itself. Illness may be caused by internal or external forces. Some believe that an individual unable to control such internal forces as anger, fright, and jealousy is susceptible to disease (Henderson & Primeaux, 1981). Illness caused by external forces are explained as the gods' way of punishing a person for his or her present sins or those committed in a previous life. Other external forces capable of causing illness are spirits of dead ancestors, powers of jealous living relatives, and various demons and spirits empowered by evildoers. Charms, medals, and trinkets may be worn to help ward off evil (Boyle & Andrews, 1989; Miller & Supersad, 1991).

In addition to acceptance of modern or Western medicine, East Indian Americans tend to believe in several highly developed health and illness systems based on complex folk beliefs and practices: the Ayurvedic, Unani, and homeopathic health theories (Nyrop, 1975).

The Ayurvedic belief system stems from ancient Hindu religion and philosophy. The Hindu medical arts were first expounded in the sacred scriptures, the Vedas. One portion of the Vedas, the Atharva-Veda, represents the popular religious faith and superstitions of the masses, which differ from the more advanced beliefs of the priestly classes. Ayurvedic medicine derived its name from the section of the Athara-Veda known as the Ayur-Veda (or Knowledge of Long Life). Ayurvedic practitioners are called *vaids* (Nyrop, 1975). The Ayurvedic system is based on the belief that disease is caused by the imbalance of essential body elements. Some East Indians acknowledge three fundamental elements of the human body—*dasa*, *dhatu*, and *mala*—which must be in a state of balance to maintain equilibrium or optimal health. *Dasa* directs the physiological functions of the body, *dhatu* is the basic structure of the human cell, and *mala* constitutes products of metabolism (Kakar, 1977). Within the Ayurvedic system, diseases are believed to be of psychosomatic origin and are treated accordingly (Dash, 1974). Most Ayurvedic medications, extracted from plants, are herbal remedies. To maintain or reestablish balance, diet is an important consideration in the therapeutic regime (Miller & Supersad, 1991).

The Unani health belief system was introduced by the Muslims. Its local practitioners are called *hakims*. Unani, which uses herbal remedies from every known plant, is similar to the Ayurvedic system.

The homeopathic health belief system has no religious affiliation. It was introduced by a German doctor in 1796. Homeopathic medicine is based on the law of similars. The theory states that minute dosages of a drug that would produce similar symptoms in a healthy person can be used to treat the diseased person. Vaccination and inoculation to produce immunity are frequently offered in support of the homeopathy theory (Nyrop, 1975).

Traditionally and in rural India today, health beliefs and practices are frequently derived from the family, in-laws (especially the mother-in-law), other elders of the community, midwives, folk practitioners, and community health workers. Therapeutic advice is usually obtained from a variety of sources on a hierarchy of five different levels:

1. The family. The mother-in-law, who assumes the role of the family health practitioner, is regarded as an authority on diagnosis and therapy.
2. Consultation of a holy man (*sanyasis*), if deemed necessary by the mother-in-law.
3. The caste level. Two or more *sanyasis* may administer to the needs of their caste members.
4. The village level. The village religious faith healer offers services free of charge, regardless of caste.
5. Consultations beyond the village from a variety of folk practitioners, including exorcists and spirit mediums (Miller & Supersad, 1991).

Andhra pradesh toddy is a tonic given to expectant mothers in the amount of about 1 liter daily. This tonic, generally prescribed by the elders, is believed to stimulate a healthy pregnancy but has actually been found to precipitate "vitamin B deficiency, sore tongue and mouth membranes, and tingling of muscles" (Raman, 1988, p. 144).

CULTURAL DIETARY PRACTICES

The preparation of an Indian meal is time-consuming. Onions must be ground to a paste, often by hand. Most Indian dishes have a base of an onion spice mixture browned in oil. Meat, vegetables, and water are added to this browned mixture and cooked until tender. Curry is a popular mixture of typical Indian spices added to gravy, which turns the food a yellowish-green. Other spices commonly used in Indian cookery are turmeric, ginger, tamarind, garlic, and coriander (Patibandla, 1994).

Most Hindus are vegetarians. Those who to eat meat do not eat beef. Muslims do not eat pork. Meat curry dishes are frequently made from goat meat or chicken.

Most East Indian Americans eat rice daily, often with *dal*, a bowl of lentil soup. Those from southern India like the hot and spicy *sambar*, a *dal* eaten with thin rice flour pancakes.

A popular bread is *roti*, which is a flat pancake like bread, prepared on a black iron griddle. One type of *roti* is prepared by dropping balls of dough into boiling oil, where they become puffy. These puffed-up roti are enjoyed on festive occasions with *halwa* (a sweet cereal).

Chapatis are a form of *roti* made of whole wheat flour, salt, butter or margarine, and water, usually baked on a heavy iron convex griddle or an earthen stove (a *chulha*). When chapatis are stuffed with grated vegetables and fried in oil, the dish is called *parata* and is often served with yogurt, which is a favorite milk dish. Another favorite dish is *panir*, a homemade cheese, which may be cut up into small pieces, deep fried, and then curried with peas and potatoes. Alcohol is forbidden to Muslims but not to Hindus; nevertheless, the latter rarely serve alcoholic beverages (Sarin, 1985).

Some East Indians, especially in rural areas, prefer to eat their food with their hands while sitting cross-legged on the floor. They wrap a piece of *roti* around meat or vegetable, dip it in *dal*, gravy, or sauce, and thus convey it to the mouth, (Sarin, 1985). The right hand is used for feeding oneself; the left hand is reserved for toileting procedures (Nyrop, 1986).

MORBIDITY AND MORTALITY

Some East Indian Americans have a genetic predisposition to thalassemia (Cooley's anemia) and lactose intolerance (Miller & Supersad, 1991). A study performed in the United Kingdom revealed that South Asians (Indians, Pakistanis, and Bangladeshis) averaged a lower alcohol consumption rate than the native British population. However, in spite of the lower consumption, alcohol morbidity rates for some South Asian communities were higher than the general population. Alcohol consumption rates were found to be higher in Sikhs than in Hindus or Muslims (McKeigue & Karmi, 1993).

Another British study of adult Asian patients revealed a notable proportion of metabolic bone disease. Osteomalacia, most prevalent in Hindu women, was associated with a strict vegetarian diet and the covering of skin when outdoors (Finch, Ang, Eastwood & Maxwell, 1992). *Chapatis*, the staple bread in some East Indian communities, is known to have a high concentration of phytate, which may decrease calcium absorption in the small intestine. Vitamin D levels appear lower in individuals who consume *chapatis* (Freimer, Echenberg & Kretchmer, 1983).

BELIEFS ABOUT DEATH AND DYING

Many Hindus perceive death as a passing from one existence to another. A person's lifespan is similar to a bead on a necklace where the other beads represent other lifetimes. Each person strives through rebirths to ascend the scale of merit to achieve union with Brahma.

Outward displays of grief (wailing, crying, chanting, and fainting) are accepted practices among family and friends. Grieving Hindu men and women are not stoic, but highly expressive. Cremation of the body is preferred (Miller & Supersad, 1991).

PHYSICAL ASSESSMENT

East Indian–American complexions range from white to olive-toned to dark brown, with hair that is generally straight or curly, except among some communities in the South, where complexions are darker. East Indians tend to have smaller frames and are generally thinner than Westerners (Nyrop, 1986).

REFERENCES

Aris, H. (1990, April 11). View from the East. *Nursing Times, 86*(15), 44–45.

Bhargava, G. (1988). Seeking immigration through matrimonial alliance: A study of advertisements in an ethnic weekly. *Journal of Comparative Family Studies, 19*(2), 245–57.

Boyle, J. S., & Andrews, M. M. (1989). *Transcultural concepts in nursing care.* Glenview, IL: Scott, Foresman.

Bureau of the Census. (1992). *Statistical abstract of the United States.* Washington, D.C.: Government Printing Office.

Chandras, K. (1977). *Arab, Armenian, Syrian, Lebanese, East Indian, Pakistani and Bangladeshi Americans: A study guide and source book.* San Francisco: R&E Research Associates.

Chekki, D. (1988). Family in India and North America: Change and continuity among Lingayat families. *Journal of Comparative Family Studies, 19*(2), 329–43.

Dash, V. B. (1974). *Ayurvedic treatment for common disease.* Delhi, India: Delhi Diary.

Dhruvarajan, V. (1988). Religious ideology and interpersonal relationships within the family. *Journal of Comparative Family Studies, 19*(2), 273–85.

Driver, E. D., & Driver, A. E. (1988). Social and demographic correlates of consanguineous marriages in South India. *Journal of Comparative Family Studies, 19*(2), 229–43.

Finch, P. J., Ang, L., Eastwood, J. B., & Maxwell, J. D. (1992). Clinical and histological spectrum of osteomalacia among Asians in south London. *Quarterly Journal of Medicine, 83*(302), 439–48.

Fishlock, T. (1983). *Gandhi's children*. New York: Universe Books.

Freimer, N., Echenberg, D., & Kretchmer, N. (1983). Cultural variation: Nutritional and clinical implications. *Western Journal of Medicine, 139*(6), 928–33.

Government Publication of India. (1993). *India, a dynamic democracy*. External Publicity Division, Ministry of External Affairs, Government of India, New Delhi.

Henderson, G., & Primeaux, M. (1981). *Transcultural health care*. Reading, MA: Addison-Wesley.

Indian Consulate General Information Section. (1991, March). *United Nations*. New York.

Jee, H. H. (1981). *Aryan medical science: A short history*. Delhi, India: Maharaja of Gundal.

Jensen, J. M. (1980). East Indians. In S. Thernstrom (Ed.), *Harvard encyclopedia of American ethnic groups* (pp. 298–301). Cambridge: Belknap Press of Harvard University Press.

Kakar, D. (1977). *Folk and modern medicine*. New Delhi: New Asian Publishers.

Kakar, D. N., Chopra, S., Samuel, S. A., & Sangar, K. (1989). Beliefs and practices related to disposal of human placenta. *Nursing Journal of India 80*(12), 315–17.

Kamar, P. (1994, January). Interview with Pavankumar Kamar, Embassy of India, Washington, D.C.

McKeigue, P. M., & Karmi, G. (1993). Alcohol consumption and alcohol related problems in Afro-Caribbeans and south Asians in the United Kingdom. *Alcohol-Alcohol, 28*(1), 1–10.

Miller, S. W., & Supersad, J. N. (1991). East Indian Hindu Americans. In J. N. Giger & R. L. Davidhizar (Eds.), *Transcultural nursing: Assessment and intervention* (pp. 436–62). St. Louis: Mosby Year Book.

Nyrop, R. F. (1986). *India: A country study*. Foreign Area Studies. Washington, DC: American University.

Nyrop, R. F. (1975). *Area handbook for India*. Foreign Area Studies. Washington, DC: American University.

Patibandla, Rao Srinivasa. (1994, January). Interview.

Peck, M. F. (1981). The therapeutic effect of faith. *Nursing Forum, 22*(2), 153.

Rajamani, J. (1994, January). Interview.

Ratnaraj, M. (1994, January). Interview.

Sarin, A. V. (1985). *India, an ancient land, a new nation*. Minneapolis: Dillon Press.

6

Filipino Americans

The Philippines, named after Prince Philip of Spain, is the oldest former colonial country in Southeast Asia. The land area forms an archipelago of about 7,000 islands located in the Pacific Ocean, 450 miles off the southeastern coast of China. The Philippines cover a total land area that is smaller than Japan, approximately the size of Arizona, and slightly larger than the United Kingdom. The archipelago has a longer coastline than that of the United States.

The archpelago can be divided into three major areas: Mindanao, Luzon, and the Visayan Islands. Mindanao, the largest, is located at the southernmost part of the archipelago and is the historical Muslim center. Luzon is the large northern island on which Manila, the largest city, is located. Between these two large islands is a group of smaller ones, known as the Visayan Islands. Parts of the Visayas, especially the island of Cebu, are the most densely populated areas of the islands, from which a significant number of Filipinos have migrated to the United States (Aquino, 1981; Melendy, 1980; Nelson, 1968).

Because of the Philippines' proximity to the equator, the islands enjoy a monsoon climate. Temperatures range from 60–90 degrees F, with a mean of 80 degrees throughout the year.

POPULATION IN THE UNITED STATES

Filipinos, numbering 1.47 million, representing 0.6% of the American population, are the second largest Asian-American population (after Chinese Americans). Within the United States, 70.5% of the Filipino population resides in the

West, 11.3% in the South, 10.2% in the Northeast, 8.1% in the Midwest, and 16.9% in Hawaii (Bureau of the Census, 1992).

Filipinos represent different cultural and linguistic groups as a result of varied migrations to the Philippines and consequent mixing of ethnic and racial groups. Filipinos have diverse origins. The Negritos were probably the first settlers to arrive in the Philippines, believed to have crossed the land bridges that connected the archipelago to Asia in 20,000 B.C. Negritos are short, brown skinned, with Negroid features. Brown-skinned Filipinos are their ancestors and are the predominant population of the Philippines (Aquino, 1981).

Other nationalities represented in peoples of the Philippines are Malaysians from southeastern Asia, Indonesians from East India, and Muslims (from the Muhammedan invasion in the fourteenth century). Chinese, Japanese, Spaniards, and Americans are also represented in the Filipino population (Affonso, 1978; Vance, 1991).

IMMIGRATION

Filipinos migrated to the United States in three distinct increments. The earliest immigrants came as students after the Spanish-American War when the Treaty of Paris in 1899 transferred imperial control of the islands from Spain to the United States. Many students returned to the Philippines, but some stayed and established communities, mainly in Hawaii and California.

The second wave, in the 1920s and early 1930s, consisted of farmworkers, essentially all males, who filled the jobs that the Chinese and Japanese had pioneered. At this time in California, Filipino men outnumbered the women 15 to 1. Filipino Americans suffered constant discrimination because, like other immigrants, they were perceived as a threat to jobs held by Americans since they were willing to accept low wages. They were also discriminated against because they were nonwhite. After World War II, the image of the Philippines greatly improved because they had served the United States as a loyal ally against the Japanese. Consequently, America granted the Philippines independence after the war in 1946 (Daniels, 1990; Melendy, 1980).

The third influx of Filipinos has come since 1965, when immigration laws became more lenient. The more recent Filipino migrants have been mostly female (Daniels, 1990).

COMMUNICATION

Filipino Americans speak over 80 different dialects. In the United States, most Filipinos speak Visayan, Tagalog (Pilipino), or Ilocano. Tagalog, the language of central Luzon, was renamed Pilipino (pronounced Filipino) in 1946 when it was proclaimed the national language. Ilocano is the language most commonly spoken by Filipinos in Hawaii and on the U.S. mainland (Melendy, 1980).

Translations of some common expressions are included at the end of this chapter.

Filipino Americans of Spanish origin might prefer a space zone that is somewhat personal (18 inches to 4 feet), whereas Filipinos of Asian descent are usually more comfortable with a wider space zone (4 to 6 feet), especially when communicating with strangers (Giger & Davidhizar, 1990).

Some Filipinos of Asian descent tend to avoid sustained eye contact. This is more pronounced between members of the opposite sex. Also some individuals are not prone to unnecessary touching. Usually affectionate touch is not practiced among strangers (Vance, 1991).

SOCIOECONOMIC STATUS

Since 1965 Filipino immigrants generally have been well educated, upwardly mobile professionals and potential entrepreneurs. About two-thirds of the recent Filipino immigrants are professionals (Daniels, 1990). Notable among these professionals are nurses and other health care personnel. Many American urban hospitals recruit Filipino nurses, who have become essential to the functioning of many major public hospitals (Daniels, 1990).

CHIEF COMPLAINT

Filipinos of Asian origin usually do not describe pain with the expected emotion because they tend to be stoic. On the other hand, Filipinos of Spanish origin may describe pain dramatically, with gestures and facial grimaces.

FAMILY

The Filipino-American family may be matriarchal or patriarchal. The father is generally the major authority figure. Grandparents also hold positions of authority within the family (Aquino, 1981). In the Philippines, families may be either nuclear or extended but more often are extended. Nuclear Filipino families are more common in the United States. Although the nuclear Filipino-American family is the basic socioeconomic unit, this family is actually a subunit of the extended kin group. It is an acceptable practice for adult unmarried employed children to live with parents in the nuclear family and contribute to family support (Almirol, 1982). Although the Filipino heritage is a blend of various cultures, there is a strong Chinese influence on Filipino family solidarity (Vance, 1991).

Some traditional Filipino Americans believe that they are judged primarily by their loyalties to the extended family. Social status could be associated with one's capacity to improve family socioeconomic level, maintain family harmony and cohesion, and protect the honor of women kin. The kin group relationship is based on a complex system of reciprocal rights and obligations in a setting of interdependence. Loyalty and unity, which are essential to family relationships, serve to promote strong ties between kin that can be advantageous. On the other hand, these strong ties tend to isolate some Filipino Americans socially from other Americans (Almirol, 1982).

Various relationships characterize the traditional Filipino-American family concept (Affonso, 1978; Vance, 1991). The most common relationship is the blood bond of a bilateral kinship system (the individual's descent is acknowledged with respect to the families of both parents). It is not unusual for the mother's maiden name to be given as a child's middle name, while the surname remains that of the father's family. Each parent is considered of equal importance, and together both families provide a bilateral inheritance system (Aquino, 1981).

The second type of relationship is affinal kinship, resulting from marriage. At the wedding, the relatives of the bride are accepted by the groom, and his relatives become the bride's family.

A third type of relationship is known as the *compadrazgo* kinship. In what was originally a Roman Catholic ritual, godparents (*compadres*) selected at the time of the child's baptism serve as coparents and assume responsibility for the child's welfare thereafter. Generally the *compadres* are selected on the basis of socioeconomic status and access to power. Ideally the *padrino* (godfather) is someone to whom the godchild can go to when in need of financial or political favors. Although this role may have altered somewhat among modern Filipinos in the United States, godparents are still viewed as surrogate parents as well as active participants in the socialization and education of their godchildren. Today it is still customary to expect the godparents to assume some of the financial expenses for baptism and to give gifts at Christmas, birthdays, weddings, and family funerals, thus becoming involved in family rites of passage. Godparent obligations may include helping to finance their godchild's education and later assisting the child to find employment, build a home, and/or purchase a car (Affonso, 1978; Almirol, 1982). The *compadrazgo* system also embodies reciprocal obligations. If the godparents have no children of their own, their godchildren are expected to provide care during the godparents' illness and old age. Thus, the *compadrazgo* system extends the kinship ties of loyalty, obligations, reciprocity, and interdependence.

The fourth type of relationship, *utang na loob*, is a system of reciprocal obligations; a person must be ready to repay another's kindness by goods or services, often on demand. Kin members borrow money and exchange food and other necessities among themselves. An individual who refuses to help a relative is regarded as shameless, *walang hiya*. *Hiya* means "shame" or "losing face," and this label must be avoided at all cost. To be *walang hiya* means to be publicly condemned (Almirol, 1982).

When Filipinos migrate and are not among blood kin, often the *compadrazgo* and/or the *utang* systems can increase their allies and provide support in adjusting to a new environment (Affonso, 1978). Most kin members who migrate to the United States are assisted by resident relatives in a system of chain migration, which means that previous immigrants may provide transportation, initial accommodations, and employment arrangements for newly arriving relatives (Almirol, 1982).

ELDERLY

Filipino-American elders are highly respected by all family members. In the Filipino culture, a nurse would not address a Filipino elderly client by the first name. The expression *po* (similar to the English *madam* and *sir*) should be used when speaking to an elder, because it conveys respect (Vance, 1991).

Children are taught to respect their elders. An important Filipino practice is that of kissing the hand of the elderly person as a sign of respect and reverence. In greeting the elder, the right hand is kissed with the words, *"mano po."* The elder may then reply with "God bless you" (Affonso, 1978).

MATERNITY CUSTOMS AND CHILD REARING

Filipino women in Hawaii and the United States tend to practice early prenatal care. Regular check-ups, exercise, a balanced diet, and good hygiene are prime considerations during pregnancy. Many believe that overeating should be avoided. Some foods are restricted during pregnancy because of traditional beliefs—for example, crabs because they will cause the baby to have clubbed fingers or toes, and dark foods like prunes and black coffee because they will produce a dark-skinned baby. A traditional belief has been that all the pregnant woman's food cravings should be immediately satisfied or the baby could be premature or have a birthmark (Affonso, 1978). Traditional beliefs perpetuate some taboos—for example, sitting on steps or standing in a doorway could block passage of the baby's head, arguing with relatives could result in complications or miscarriage, and walking over a rope could result in a delayed expulsion of the placenta.

Some Filipino-American mothers massage their newborn baby with oil and dress the child in white. Traditionally white has been preferred for baby clothing because white symbolizes the purity that God has bestowed on newborns. Some traditional practices are thought to maintain the health of the newborn: daily washing, massaging, and oiling the baby to protect the delicate skin and stimulate muscle growth; placing a fifty-cent piece on the umbilicus secured by a belly band, to promote proper healing; attaching a religious medal to the baby's clothing to keep the child safe; avoid exposing the infant to bright colors to prevent strabismus; and keeping garlic and salt near the baby at all times to ward off evil spirits (Affonso 1978).

In the traditional Filipino-American family, sex is considered a delicate subject and is seldom discussed openly. Boys may be circumcised during adolescence, although the procedure varies depending on the community and prevailing practices. Traditional Filipino-American parents are generally authoritarian and strict. They teach their children the importance of conformity and avoidance of shame or disgrace to the family. Children are expected to practice respectful, obedient and humble behavior in their daily life. Education is highly valued (Affonso, 1978; Vance, 1991).

SOCIALIZATION PATTERNS

Filipino Americans generally have mild, passive temperaments. They tend to place great importance on balance and harmony in social interactions and seldom express disagreement, especially with those in authority. They are usually quiet, polite, respectful of authority, and able to suppress outward hostility. Anger may be dealt with in a passive-aggressive manner using behavior manifestations such as procrastination, stubbornness, desire for acceptance, and various attention-seeking tactics (Aquino, 1981; DeGracia, 1979; Vance, 1991).

A basic value held by some Filipino Americans is *pakikisama*, which means maintaining good feelings in all personal interactions and being able to get along with others at all costs. Social acceptance is extremely important. Filipino Americans may tend to agree even when they mistrust the physician or nurse to avoid hurting the other person's feelings. Generally Filipinos prefer not to disagree with those in authority. Health professionals are considered people in authority. Some Filipino men may experience discomfort in the presence of a female authority figure (Vance, 1991).

In a study of family life, Pullium (1988) found that, in contrast to the belief that the self-esteem of Asian women is elevated by having a large family, the Filipino-American mother's self-esteem was positively related to her educational level rather than her family size. Actually, family size tended to show a negative relationship to self-esteem, and the number of children also had a negative effect on parental satisfaction, children's education, and family health (Pullium, 1988).

RELIGIOUS BELIEFS AND PRACTICES

Throughout the Spanish colonial period (1521–1898), the Roman Catholic church was an important political, educational, and economic power in the Philippines. Consequently, the Philippines became the only Christian nation in the Far East, and so most Filipinos are Roman Catholic (Aquino, 1981; Melendy, 1980; Vance, 1991).

CULTURALLY BASED HEALTH BELIEFS AND PRACTICES

Traditionally it has been believed that illness results when the internal and external elements of the body are disturbed. Factors that may disturb the normal equilibrium of these elements are changes in seasons, improper diet, witchcraft, accidents, and inappropriate behaviors. Some Filipino Americans say special prayers of protection, perform rituals, use holy water, and/or wear such articles as charms, medals, or crucifixes for protection against external disease agents (Aquino, 1981).

Traditional Filipino-American health beliefs and practices may be based on three concepts:

1. Flushing, the perception of the body as a container that collects and holds impurities. A common home remedy used to cause flushing is vinegar, believed to be able to flush out the system in the treatment of a cold or fever.

2. Heating practices, based on the belief that hot and cold must be kept in balance within the body. Extremes of hot and cold can cause illness.

3. Protection, to keep the body's external boundaries safe from disease and other evil forces (McKenzie & Chrisman, 1977; Vance, 1991).

Because the culture of the Philippines has been influenced by different ethnic groups—Chinese, East Indian, Arab, Spanish, and American—a variety of folk practices exist (Vance, 1991). Some folk beliefs associated with illness and health include the following:

• Combing the hair at night will cause diseases of the eye.

• Sleeping with wet hair will result in blindness.

• Bathing during menstruation will cause insanity.

• Bathing on Fridays is unhealthy.

• Large ears are an indication of longevity.

• Crucifixes, charms, or medals should be attached to the clothing of babies to protect them from evil spirits and effects of the evil eye.

• If an expectant mother takes a special fancy to the statue of the Virgin Mary, her child will be very beautiful (Aquino, 1981, p. 182).

CULTURAL DIETARY PATTERNS

Filipino Americans who believe in the hot-cold dichotomy may prepare meals by including "hot" and "cold" (unrelated to temperature) foods. For example, beans, considered "hot," are served with vegetables, considered "cold" (Orque, Bloch & Monrroy, 1983). Favorite Filipino-American foods are fish, vegetables, and rice (Rafael 1990). Typical dishes might include *adobo*, a highly seasoned, spicy dish made of pork and chicken cooked in vinegar and lard; *lumpi*, prepared with selected vegetables and similar to Chinese egg roll; and *pancit*, rice or noodles cooked with ham, chicken, or shrimps in soy and garlic sauce (Ignacio, 1976; Vance, 1991).

MORBIDITY AND MORTALITY

Thalassemia (Cooley's anemia) is prevalent among Filipinos (Vance, 1991). Filipinos of Chinese descent may exhibit a lactose intolerance (Gerber, 1983).

Filipino-American men and women have the highest rate of hypertension among the Asian population in the United States (Klatsky & Armstrong, 1991). Although they show a high prevalence rate for hypertension, they record low rates of hypertension mortality, perhaps related to appropriate control practices, knowledge of risk factors, and behavior modification. Filipino Americans demonstrate a lower risk for cigarette smoking and alcohol abuse than Caucasians (Stavig, Igra, Leonard, McCullough & Oreglia, 1986).

In Hawaii, where Filipinos constitute 20% of the population, Filipino-American women were found to have the lowest incidence of breast cancer, as compared to Japanese, Chinese, ethnic Hawaiians, and Caucasians. However, late-stage diagnosis is common among the Filipino Americans, and thus their death rate from the disease is greater than that for the other cultures (Goodman, 1991).

Asian-descent Filipino Americans tend to be less active and experience fewer accidents than Caucasians (Chung, Tash, Raymond, Yasunobu & Lew, 1990).

BELIEFS ABOUT DEATH AND DYING

Beliefs about death and dying are related to the Roman Catholic religion.

PHYSICAL ASSESSMENT

Filipinos, classed as Asians, generally have complexions that range from olive to brown, almond-shaped eyes, and sparse body hair. Hair on the head is usually coarse, straight or curly, and dark brown to black in color. Male baldness is rare (Garn, 1965; Vance, 1991). (If the client is dark-skinned, refer to the section on assessment of dark skin in Chapter 1 on African Americans.)

Filipinos are generally shorter and thinner and have smaller bone structures than their white counterparts (Meredith, 1978). Filipino babies exhibit a lower mean birth weight than white babies (Morton, 1977; Vance, 1991), so standard Western charts on growth and development may produce inaccurate impressions.

Translations of Some Common Filipino Terms

English	Filipino
Doctor	*Doktor*
Surgery	*Operasyon*
Pain	*Masakit*
Bowels	*Na*

Food (I am hungry)	*Gusto kong kumain*
Chair (I want to sit)	*Gusto kong umupo*
Bath (I want to bathe)	*Gusto kung maligo*
Voided	*Naiihi ako*
Medications	*Gamot*
Indication of gratitude	*Hiya*
Knowledge	*Karunungan*
Movement	*Kaunlaran*
Good	*Mabuti*
Hope	*Pagasa*
Bad	*Sama*
Gratitude	*Utang na loob*

Sources: Ignacio, 1976; interview with Jon Rafael, August 1990.

REFERENCES

Affonso, D. D. (1978). The Filipino American. In A. L. Clark (Ed.), *Culture, childbearing health professionals* (pp. 128–53). Philadelphia: F. A. Davis Company.

Almirol, E. B. (1982). Rights and obligations in Filipino American families. *Journal of Comparative Family Studies, 13*(3), 291–306.

Aquino, C. J. (1981). The Filipino in America. In A. L. Clark (Ed.), *Culture and child-rearing* (pp. 166–90). Philadelphia: F. A. Davis Company.

Bureau of the Census. (1992). *Statistical abstracts of the United States.* Washington, DC: Government Printing Office.

Chung, C. S., Tash, E., Raymond, J., Yasunobu, C., & Lew, R. (1990). Health risk behaviors and ethnicity in Hawaii. *International Journal of Epidemiology, 19*(4), 1011–18.

Daniels, R. (1990). *Coming to America: A history of immigration and ethnicity in American life.* Princeton, NJ: HarperCollins.

DeGracia, R. T. (1979, August). Cultural influences on Filipino patients. *American Journal of Nursing*, 1412–14.

Garn, S. (1965). *Human races* (2d ed.) Springfield, IL: Charles C. Thomas.

Gerber, L. M. (1983). Gains in life experience of heart disease and stroke were eliminated among Caucasians, Filipinos and Japanese in Hawaii. *Social Science and Medicine, 17*(6), 349–53.

Giger, J. N., & Davidhizar, R. (1990, January–February). Transcultural nursing assessment: A method for advancing nursing practice. *International Nursing Review, 37*(1), 199–202.

Goodman, M. J. (1991). Breast cancer in multi-ethnic populations: The Hawaii perspective. *Breast Cancer Research and Treatment, 18*(1), 85–89.

Ignacio, L. F. (1976). *Asian American and Pacific Islanders: Is there such an ethnic group?* San Jose, CA: Pilipino Development Associates.

Klatsky, A. L., & Armstrong, M. A. (1991). Cardiovascular risk factors among Asian

Americans living in northern California. *American Journal of Public Health,*
81(11), 1423–28.

McKenzie, J., & Chrisman, N. (1977). Healing herbs, gods and magics. *Nursing Outlook,*
25, 326–28.

Melendy, H. B. (1977). *Asians in America: Filipinos, Koreans, and East Indians.* Boston:
Twayne Publishers.

Melendy, H. B. (1980). Filipinos. In S. Thernstrom (Ed.), *Harvard encyclopedia of Amer-*
ican ethnic groups (pp. 354–62). Cambridge: Belknap Press of Harvard University
Press.

Meredith, H. (1978). Research between 1960 and 1970 on the standing heights of young
children in different parts of the world. In H. Reese & L. Lipsitt (Eds.), *Advances*
in child development and behavior (pp. 1–59). New York: Academic Press.

Nelson, R. (1968). *The Philippines.* New York: Walker and Company.

Orque, M. S., Bloch, B., & Monrroy, L. S. A. (1983). *Ethnics in nursing care: A mul-*
ticultural approach. St. Louis: C. V. Mosby.

Pullium, R. M. (1988, Spring). What makes good families: Predictors of family welfare
in the Philippines. *Journal of Comparative Family Studies, 20*(1), 47–66.

Raman, A. V. (1988). Traditional practices and nutritional taboos. *The Nursing Journal*
of India, 79(6), 143–45, 166.

Stavig, G. R., Igra, A., Leonard, A. R., McCullough, J., & Oreglia, A. (1986). Hyperten-
sion-related mortality in California. *Public Health Reports, 103*(1), 28–37.

Vance, A. R. (1991). Filipino Americans. In J. N. Giger & R. E. Davidhizar (Eds.),
Transcultural nursing: Assessment and intervention (pp. 279–401). St. Louis:
Mosby Year Book.

Watkins, D., & Astilla, E. (1979). Self-esteem and social class in the Philippines. *Journal*
of Psychology, 102(2), 211–14.

7

German Americans

Germany, located in the heart of Europe, is entirely surrounded by land except for the Baltic Sea on the northeast and the North Sea on the northwest. Between the seas, Germany is adjacent to Denmark on the north. In clockwise order beginning on the east, Germany is bordered by Poland, the Czech Republic, Austria, Switzerland, Luxembourg, Belgium, and the Netherlands. Germany has many rivers. The chief and best loved are the Rhine and the Danube. The German climate is temperate but quite changeable. In the winter months, temperatures range from about 24 to 38 degrees F; in the spring and fall, about 48 to 64 degrees F; and during the summer months, about 70 to 78 degrees F (Cussans & Peterson, 1991; Peck, 1970).

Beginning on January 30, 1933, Hitler was Germany's chancellor for 12 years. After his death at the end of World War II, Germany was divided into East and West Zones by the Soviets and the other Allies. In 1949, Soviet forces occupied East Germany and called the area the German Democratic Republic (GDR); the United States managed the Federal Republic or West Germany (Asmus, 1990; Halliday, 1990; Myer & Breslau, 1990; Nemeth, 1990).

On October 3, 1990, the fall of the Berlin wall heralded the reunification of Germany. Berlin's status as a free city presented both advantages and disadvantages. Because of the current influx of people to Germany, city officials predict that the population will double to about 6 million by the year 2015 and that Berlin will again become one of the most vibrant cities in Europe. However, East Berlin has had serious financial problems and its communist officials in the past were inflexible and unaccustomed to assuming initiative (Meyer, 1990).

POPULATION IN THE UNITED STATES

German Americans number approximately 60 million individuals, representing 23.3% of the American population (Bureau of the Census, 1992). Early waves of German immigrants settled in Pennsylvania, the Carolinas, Texas, Missouri, Minnesota, and particularly Wisconsin. The earlier generations preferred to settle in the rural areas; later immigrants concentrated in major cities, among them New York (port of entry), Milwaukee, Cincinnati, Buffalo, St. Louis, Chicago, Cleveland, Toledo, Dayton, and Detroit, where they attempted to replicate the culture of their homeland. Some referred to a German triangle, with St. Louis, Cincinnati, and Milwaukee as the three points (Daniels, 1990).

IMMIGRATION

Germans began migrating to the United States in the seventeenth century for economic, political, or religious reasons. During the peak immigration years, between the 1830s and the 1880s, Germans were never less than one-quarter of all immigrants. Between 1880 and 1920, they represented the largest first-generation immigrant population in America. The early waves of German immigrants were described as industrious, frugal, and skilled farmers who were more concerned with their land and livestock than with their own personal comfort. Their persistence, discipline, and mutual aid brought them prosperity, although few were notably wealthy during the colonial period (Conzen, 1980; Daniels, 1990).

Some German Americans migrated to escape the political revolutions that spread through Europe during 1848. These immigrants were known as the Forty-eighters. Unlike their predecessors, who were on the whole politically apathetic, the Forty-eighters excelled in politics and military skills. One vociferous spokesman for the Forty-eighters was Carl Schurz. Along with others from this group who achieved outstanding military recognition, Schurz became a distinguished Union general in the Civil War. He then went on to become a U.S. senator from Missouri and later secretary of the interior. The Forty-eighters opposed slavery, favored preserving the Union, and consequently played a significant role in the winning of the Civil War (Rippley, 1970; Winawer-Steiner & Wetzel, 1982).

The last significant immigration wave after 1848 was referred to as the intellectuals' migration. These well-educated and highly skilled refugees, fleeing Hitler, were generally older than the previous immigrant groups. Their intent was to share their knowledge; as one German scholar expressed, "Think of what you can give to America, not what you can get out of her" (Rippley, 1970, p. 54). Among these intellectual Germans were Albert Einstein and Thomas Mann (Winawer-Steiner & Wetzel, 1982).

German Jews in America maintained both their German and Jewish heritages. Besides religion, they differed from other Germans in various respects. Characteristically, they demonstrated a lower return migration to Germany than did other Germans. They were seldom farmers and thus often preferred to settle in the cities, where they were attracted to tailoring and the retail trade. Some established retail and wholesale establishments that became well known, such as Sears Roebuck, Rich's in Atlanta, and Sakowitz in Houston (Daniels, 1990). (Chapter 12, on Jewish Americans, contains a discussion of German Jews.)

COMMUNICATION

German is the language spoken. Translation of some German expressions are presented at the end of this chapter.

German Americans seldom use emotional overtones in their speech. During communication some German Americans tend to prefer a wide space zone, are unlikely to touch others, and may react negatively when touched (Giger & Davidhizar, 1990).

SOCIOECONOMIC STATUS

During the late nineteenth century, German-born women were less likely to be found in the industrial labor force than were other immigrant or native-born American women. Those German-American women who did work outside the home seemed to prefer the service sectors. They were most frequently bakers, domestic workers, laundry workers and saloon keepers but seldom factory or clerical workers. In the early years, domestic work for women served a dual purpose: it provided funds to help the household and exposed these immigrants to American middle-class home life, which helped promote their acculturation and assimilation (Daniels, 1990).

Home ownership was more prevalent among German Americans than among other groups of similar socioeconomic status. In Missouri and western Illinois, the typical German cottage, built up to the street line and having a garden in the back, is still a familiar sight. Distinctive brickwork of German tradition still exists in some old homes and churches (Conzen, 1980).

Results of a study by Ott (1990) conducted in West Germany indicated that although socioeconomic factors influence life-style, education is the best predictor of behavior (more so than income or occupation). In West Germany, education is the major factor that influences behavior in favor of a healthy life-style.

CHIEF COMPLAINT

German Americans may not describe symptoms with the expected emotion. They tend to be stoic and reluctant to complain. Some Germans tend to be quite independent and are less willing than individuals of some other cultures to play the sick role (Bischoff, 1987). Traditional German Americans prefer to avoid doctors if possible (Wittmann, 1991).

FAMILY

The German-American family type is usually patriarchal and nuclear, with the husband/father the undisputed head and leader of the family. He is the dominant authority figure, and his wife and children are subordinate to him. The father's responsibility is to provide for the family's material needs by hard work. He handles the family finances, does all repairs around the house, and is responsible for the upkeep of the family car. He has the right to make all major decisions unilaterally or to ratify any decisions made by the couple. Some Germans have described the father as an authoritarian and stern tyrant and the mother as warm, loving, and subservient (Winawer-Steiner & Wetzel, 1982).

The early Pennsylvania Germans (Pennsylvania Dutch) accepted the male dominant social order. The women directed their lives by the old trinity: *Kinder, Kirche, Kuche* (children, church, kitchen), while the men were involved with the farm, the mill and economic enterprises (Parsons, 1976; Rippley, 1970).

In contemporary German-American families, the wife's main task is the housework. She takes great pride in an immaculately clean house, as well as children and a husband who are neat and clean in appearance. She is usually more involved with the children than her husband, who may be somewhat emotionally distant from them. German women are often perceived as strong and hardy and capable of strenuous work (Conzen, 1980).

CHILD REARING

Traditional Concepts

In traditional Germany, bearing children has been associated with a number of folk beliefs:

- Rocking an empty cradle will bring a sleepless baby.
- The unborn baby's heart will be burned out if the pregnant mother consumes alcoholic beverages.
- It is lucky to be born after midnight but not on April 1, believed to be the birthday of Judas.
- Plant a tree (*Lebensbaum*) at the birth of a son, and the fate of the tree will coincide with the fate of the child in life.
- Throwing the placenta at the foot of a newly planted tree along with water and mother's milk will ensure fertility and happiness.

- The mother is considered impure after childbirth and should be cleansed by receiving the benediction or *Vorsegnung* in church about six weeks postpartum.

- Baptism should be planned to take place as soon as possible, not later than three months after birth, when the godparents are selected. It is believed that the child will take after the *Pate* or *Gevatter* (godfather), who should be carefully selected (Rippley, 1970).

Modern Concepts

The West German birth rate is the lowest in the world. There are few families with more than one or two children (Brand, 1989). Factors such as increasing educational achievement and greater independence of women in West Germany have apparently influenced the trend toward later marriages (in early 30s) and women having children at a later age than in previous years (Blossfeld & Jaen-ichen, 1992).

Generally German-American infants and children are raised in environments that provide more structure and spatial limitation than in mainstream American homes (Winawer-Steiner & Wetzel, 1982). The early German refugees were critical of the typical American child-centered home. Their authoritarian, patri-archal families viewed this practice as "American softness" (Rippley, 1970, p. 52). Thus, German-American child rearing reflected a concern for structure, and parents tended to be more controlling than their American counterparts.

German-American parents are perceived as being very strict, allowing their children little autonomy. The overall family atmosphere focuses more on tasks and accomplishments than on nurturing and emotions. Many German-American children are expected to be polite, show appropriate table manners, and perform their household tasks. Some families do not encourage the children to express their emotions freely (Winawer-Steiner & Wetzel, 1982). Family disagreements between parents and children are often handled autocratically, with final decisions made by the father or parents. If there is a family dispute that cannot be resolved, adult children may move out and disconnect in a process referred to as individuation and continuing relatedness. Some German-American family members have been known to sever all contact with each other rather than reconcile their differences (Stierlin, Rucker-Emboden, Wetzel & Wirsching, 1980).

Similar to some other cultures, German-American mothers are concerned with their children beginning to learn as early as possible. The kindergarten was introduced in the United States by Friedrich Froebel (Rippley, 1970), although another source has attributed the first kindergarten to Margaretha Schurz, wife of the famous German Forty-eighter, Carl Schurz (Winawer-Steiner & Wetzel, 1982). Germans made a major impact on American graduate education with the founding of Johns Hopkins University in 1876, the first institution to require a bachelor's degree for admission. All of the founding faculty were either German or held doctorates from German universities. Thus German Americans have significantly influenced the extremes of the American educational system: kindergarten and graduate school.

SOCIALIZATION PATTERNS

Some German Americans prefer to have everything in order, as expressed by a popular phrase, *Alles in Ordnung*. Other phases confirm this practice—for example: *Erst besinnen, dann beginnen* ("First think, then begin"); *Heilige Ordnung, segensreiche Himmelstochter* ("Holy order, the richly blessed daughter of heaven"), and *Ordung ist das halbe Leben* ("Order is half of life") (Rippley, 1970, p. 72). A major cultural theme is order (*Ordnung*), which is related to the management and control of the body and the realization that society is embodied in the person (Karin, 1991).

Another characteristic of the German heritage is emotional restraint. Usually affection, anger, and other emotions are not readily expressed. Many German Americans are not prone to demonstrate emotional behavior. Frequently, passions may be repressed or vented in literature and the arts. German literature and the music of the great German masters manifest this ability to sublimate emotions into art forms. Another acceptable form of expression for Germans is noted in the tradition of *Gemütlichkeit*, roughly defined as geniality, comfort, and warmth, as related to family life and pleasant social situations (Daniels, 1990).

Some German-American characteristics are thoroughness, diligence, industriousness, and craftsmanship with a keen attention to detail. Many modern German Americans tend to be perfectionists, and work success has a major impact on their self-esteem (Winawer-Steiner and Wetzel, 1982). German-American homes tend to be immaculate because of a strong focus on cleanliness and orderliness (Daniels, 1990).

The tavern is often the center of social activity in German-American neighborhoods, serving as the meeting place for clubs and German men after work. Beautifully landscaped summer beer gardens are the sites of public feasts, music, dancing, singing, and festivities for the entire family. Many recreational activities are enhanced by a glass of beer, wine, or schnapps (Conzen, 1980). Although fine wines are enjoyed, beer is the favorite German drink, with Germans ranking number one in the world for beer consumption (Cockerham, Kunz & Lueschen, 1988).

RELIGIOUS BELIEFS AND PRACTICES

Most German Americans are Protestants, the most numerous of which are Lutherans. Methodist and Unitarians represent a small number. In addition, about a third are Roman Catholic, and a sizable number are Jews (Daniels, 1990).

CULTURALLY BASED HEALTH BELIEFS AND PRACTICES

Among traditional health beliefs are the following:

- If possible, avoid doctors.
- Treat a sore throat by wrapping the neck with a wool scarf for warmth.
- Teas and other special herbal mixtures are healing remedies for throat and stomach conditions.
- Wet packs (hot and cold) can relieve aches and pains.
- Pure air and water promote good health.
- After eating fruit, do not drink water for at least one hour, in order to prevent a stomachache.
- Treat chest congestion by rubbing the chest with goose grease and wrapping it in flannel.

There is a strong belief that most illnesses are related to problems with circulation, and circulatory disturbance, *Krieslausftorung*, is a popular diagnosis (Hayes, 1991; Wittmann, 1991).

Generally German Americans are illness-prevention oriented. Mineral waters for drinking, bathing, and inhaling are often used for their preventive and healing properties. Health resorts or spas are popular German prevention and treatment modalities. A spa may be prescribed as therapy by a physician in Germany. For example, after a heart attack, a spa may be prescribed for rehabilitation and is funded by the government health insurance (Hayes, 1991; Wittmann, 1991). There are about 250 health resorts and mineral springs in Germany, of four main types: mineral spas that use warm water springs, seaside spas that rely on the therapeutic affect of seawater, hydropathic spas that employ an invigorating process, and climate health resorts, usually in the mountains, that offer health-related properties of their climate and location. Although these spas are expensive, they remain popular tourist attractions (Cussans & Peterson, 1991).

One study (Cockerham, Kunz & Lueschen, 1988a) compared life-styles in the United States and West Germany in order to ascertain whether people without the security of a government-sponsored health insurance plan put more effort into staying healthy than those who have ready access to such a program. Overall they found no significant differences in health life-styles between West German and American individuals. Yet it was noted that West Germans were more likely to drink alcohol, select healthy foods, and take time to relax, whereas Americans were more likely to emphasize physical appearance, to exercise, and to rate their health more positively. For both Germans and Americans, the better-educated individuals participated more in exercise and sports and selected healthier diets.

A subsequent study by Cockerham, Kunz, and Lueschen (1988b) found that West Germans were more likely than Americans to practice healthy eating habits. They tended to focus less on physical appearance, instead using an internal locus of control to manage their health-related dietary habits. They also worried less about their health and had a lower obesity rate than Americans. Some German Americans eat certain foods primarily for health reasons and are less narcissistic about their appearance than mainstream Americans.

CULTURAL DIETARY PATTERNS

A number of American culinary practices have German origins. The popular American delicatessen is a special German store where fine foods are sold (*Delikat* means "delicate," and *Essen* means "food"). German favorites such as sauerkraut, pumpernickel bread, and pastry are familiar to most Americans. Germans are known as great sausage eaters; the popular American hot dog is named after the German city Frankfurt. Although ground meat was named after the city of Hamburg, hamburgers appear to be an American invention and are seldom eaten by Germans (Rippley, 1970). However, this may have changed somewhat since Wendy's and McDonald's can now be found in West Germany (Cussans & Peterson, 1991).

The German sausage (*wurst*) is a popular staple found in many varieties that may be observed hanging in any German restaurant or food store: *bratwurst* for frying; brockwurst for heating in hot but not boiling water; mettwurst, katenwurst, and bierwurst to be sliced and eaten; and teewurst and leberwurst to be spread on bread. Some *wurst* varieties must be eaten fresh; others remain edible for years (Peck, 1970).

Germans like sour foods. *Sauerbraten* is beef marinated in vinegar before cooking and served with applesauce, red cabbage, and potato pancakes. German cakes, cookies, frostings, and puddings are distinctly less sweet than American desserts. Whereas the French and Belgians cook with butter and the Spanish and Italians prefer olive oil, the Germans usually cook with lard. Starches are common, and most dishes are served with noodles, dumplings, or potatoes. Although diets may include all types of breads, many Germans prefer dark breads, especially pumpernickel. Beer is the universal beverage (Cussans & Peterson, 1991).

Eating to "fill you up" may have a negative connotation to Americans because it suggests overeating. In West Germany this expression implies satisfaction and a personal sense of security and thus has a positive connotation (Cockerham, Kunz & Lueschen, 1988b). Interestingly, an earlier study (Lueschen, Guenther, Cockerham & Kunz 1987) found higher rates of obesity among Americans than among West Germans.

MORBIDITY AND MORTALITY

In a study of the incidence of disease in 2,114 individuals in Germany, diseases occurring most frequently (in declining order) were circulatory disorders, cold and influenza, vertebral disc or back conditions, high blood pressure, digestive and problems, and arthritis (Ott, 1990).

During the nineteenth century prejudices against people with disabilities, poor people, and immigrants generated the study of ''race improvement,'' called eugenics. It flourished in Nazi Germany. Some Nazi scientists and physicians designed programs of sterilization and later the extermination of people they believed were ''not worth living.'' Remembering this history, some German-American women may avoid new techniques in prenatal diagnosis because they perceive them as other ways to determine what kinds of people are fit to live (Hubbard, 1986).

BELIEFS ABOUT DEATH AND DYING

Beliefs about death and dying are related to the various religious affiliations.

Translations of Some Common German Terms

English	German
Yes	*Ja*
No	*Nein*
Nurse	*Schwester*
Doctor	*Arzt*
Thank you	*Danke schön*
Minister	*Pastor*
Rabbi	*Rabbiner*
Husband	*Mann*
Wife	*Frau*
Mother	*Mutter*
Father	*Vater*
Social worker	*Sozial-Fuersorger*
Psychologist	*Psychologist*
Pain	*Schmerzen*
Hot	*Heiss*
Cold	*Kalt*
Numb	*Erstarrt*
Hungry	*Hungrig*
Thirsty	*Durstig*
Short of breath	*Kurzatmigkeit*
Allegric	*Allergisch*
Food	*Essen*
Medicine	*Medizin*
Urinal	*Urinieren*

bedpan	*Bettschuessel*
bath	*Bad*
oxygen	*Sauerstoff*
blanket	*Bettdecke*
water	*Wasser*
coffee	*Kaffee*
Tissues	*Papiertuecher*
Dentures	*Gebiss*
money	*Geld*
Leave me alone.	*Ruhe*
No visitors	*Keine Besuche*
Get out of bed.	*Aufstehen*
Back to bed	*Zurück ins Bett*
Sit down	*Im Stuhl Sitzen*
Walk	*Gehen*
Go home	*Nach Hause Gehen*
TV	*TV*
Radio	*Radio*
On	*An*
Off	*Aus*
Change	*Wechseln*

Source: Beamatic Communicator. Courtesy of Omnimed Inc., Pine Avenue, P.O. Box 446, Maple Shade, NJ 08052-0446.

REFERENCES

Asmus, R. D. (1990, Spring). A united Germany. *Foreign Affairs, 69*(4), 63.

Bischoff, U. (1987). From Edinburgh to Berlin. *Nursing Times, 83*(35), 34–35.

Blossfeld, H., & Jaenichen, U. (1992). Educational expansion and changes in women's entry into marriage and motherhood in the Federal Republic of Germany. *Journal of Marriage and the Family, 54*(2), 302.

Brand, R. (1989). Single parents and family preservation in the Federal Republic of Germany. *Child Welfare, 68*(2), 189–95.

Bureau of the Census. (1992). *Statistical abstract of the United States.* Washington, DC: Government Printing Office.

Cockerham, W. C., Kunz, G., & Lueschen, G. (1988a, June). Social stratification and health lifestyles in two systems of health care delivery: A comparison of the United States and West Germany. *Journal of Health and Social Behavior, 29*, 113–26.

Cockerham, W. C., Kunz, G., & Lueschen, G. (1988b, September). On concern with appearance, health beliefs, and eating habits: A reappraisal comparing Americans and West Germans. *Journal of Health and Social Behavior, 29*, 265–69.

Conzen, K. N. (1980). Germans. In S. Thernstrom (Ed.), *Harvard encyclopedia of American ethnic groups* (pp. 405–25). Cambridge: Belknap Press of Harvard University Press.

Cussans, T., & Peterson, L. (1991). *Fodor's '91 Germany*. New York: Fodor's Travel Publications.

Daniels, R. (1990). *Coming to America: A history of immigration and ethnicity in American life*. Princeton, NJ: HarperCollins.

Giger, J. N., & Davidhizar, R. (1990). Transcultural nursing assessment: A method of advancing nursing practice. *International Nursing Review, 39*(1), 199–201.

Halliday, F. (1990, October 5). The final curtain: A united Germany is again the dominant European player. *New Statesman and Society, 3*(121), 10.

Hayes, D. (1991). Interview.

Hubbard, R. (1986). Eugenics and prenatal testing. *International Journal of Health Service, 16*(2), 227–42.

Karin, N. (1991). *A sound family makes a sound state: Ideology and upbringing in a German village*. Stockholm: Almqvist & Wiskell International.

Lueschen, G., Cockerham, W. C., & Kunz, G. (1987). Deutsch und amerikanische Gesundeitskultur-oder: What they say when you sneeze. *Medizin Mensch Gesellschaft, 12*, 56–69.

Meyer, M. (1990, October 8). Rebirth in Berlin: The old imperial city could become the capital of united Germany. *Newsweek*, 38–42.

Meyer, M., & Breslau, K. (1990, October 8). Day one for a new Germany. *Newsweek*, p. 45.

Nemeth, M. (1990, February 12). Uniting the Fatherland. *Maclean's, 103*(7), 30.

Ott, A. F. (1990). Life styles, job environment and health status: Some empirical findings for West Germany. *Social Science Journal, 27*(3), 339–56.

Parsons, W. F. (1976). *The Pennsylvania Dutch*. Boston: Twayne.

Peck, R. (1970). *The West Germans: How they live and work*. New York: Praeger.

Rippley, L. (1970). *Of German ways*. Minneapolis: Dillon Press.

Stierlin, H., Rucker-Embden, I., Wetzel, N., & Wirsching, M. (1980). *The first interview with the family*. New York: Brunner/Mazel.

Winawer-Steiner, H., & Wetzel, N. A. (1982). German families. In M. McGoldrick, J. K. Pearce & J. Giordano (Eds.), *Ethnicity and family therapy* (pp. 247–68). New York: Guilford Press.

Wittmann, E. (1991). Interview.

8

Haitian Americans

The small Republic of Haiti is located in the West Indies. Haiti and Dominica together constitute the island of Hispaniola among the Caribbean islands. Haiti, which is a little larger than the state of Maryland, occupies the western third of Hispaniola. Although Dominica and Haiti lie in close proximity, they are quite different culturally. Haiti is bounded by Dominica on the east, the Atlantic Ocean on the north, and the Caribbean Sea on the west and south. South America lies to the south, the island of Jamaica is to the west, and Cuba lies to the northwest of Haiti. Because Haiti is near the equator, temperatures are usually high year round. Haiti experiences a tropical climate similar to the other Caribbean islands (Chaney, 1987).

POPULATION IN THE UNITED STATES

About 290,000 Haitian Americans live in the United States, constituting 0.1% of the U.S. population (Bureau of the Census, 1992). Most Haitians have settled in New York and Florida (ports of entry). High concentrations are found in New York City, Miami, and Chicago. They tend to live in close proximity to West Indians.

In Haiti, they experience cultural and social distinctions but majority status. In the United States, they experience racism and minority status. Therefore, race, rather than culture, becomes the overriding factor of identification in American society. Haitian Americans cope with racism either by allying with African Americans or by isolating themselves through adherence to French language and culture. Haitian Americans of the latter group prefer to be called ''Frenchie'' and are determined "to stay Haitian to avoid being Black twice" (Schiller, DeWind, Brutus, Charles, Fouron & Thomas, 1987, p. 187).

IMMIGRATION

Most Haitian Americans are descendants of West African slaves brought to Haiti by France after Columbus discovered the island of Hispaniola in 1492. Through the efforts of important Haitians like Toussaint L'Ouverture, Haiti gained its freedom from France in 1804 and became the first black republic in the world. However, under the harsh dictatorship of the Duvaliers since 1957, Haiti has experienced massive oppression and poverty (Schiller et al., 1987).

Haitian Americans are a relatively new immigrant group to the United States. Haitian immigration waves did not begin until after World War II, and the major migration occurred after François Duvalier ("Papa Doc") came into power in 1957. Duvalier's political rivals and opponents, who became targets of the dictator's notorious executioners (the *ton ton macoutes*), were the first to leave. They were immediately followed by members of the elite classes, mostly mulattos who were strongly tied to international trade. These upper-class immigrants were political refugees. They spoke French, sent their children to European schools, tried to maintain French colonial practices, and generally did not associate with members of the lower economic classes. Middle-class migrants followed shortly after the elite (Schiller et al., 1987).

A second major exodus occurred when Jean-Claude Duvalier ("Baby Doc") took over power after his father's death in 1971. These immigrants, the boat people, were mainly peasants and semiskilled workers who fled from Haiti to escape poverty and political oppression. Unlike the upper socioeconomic class immigrants who were able to flee with their entire families, these poorer individuals often migrated without intact family units. They retained more African practices and spoke Creole instead of French.

Between 1967 and 1984, Haitians came to the United States from all areas of Haiti. Some held legal visas, some had student visas, and undetermined numbers became undocumented aliens. Because undocumented immigrants were considered responsible for the high unemployment rate in the United States the Immigration and Naturalization Service (INS), organized a program to detain these boat people in camps and take legal action to deport them. Numerous organizations—the Haitian Fathers, National Council of Churches, Emergency Civil Liberties Union, and the Congressional Black Caucus, among others—worked diligently to assist the boat people. In 1980, they were given entrant status, with a right to work, receive an education, and obtain financial assistance (Leavitt & Lutz, 1988).

COMMUNICATION

Creole, French, and English are the languages spoken in Haiti. Creole is spoken universally, but only a small percentage (about 2–5%) fluently speak

French, the official language and considered very prestigious. The language spoken by an individual reinforces the socioeconomic differences that separate the educated elite and growing middle class from the less educated lower class (Buchanan-Stafford, 1987).

Creole originated during the colonial period through acculturation of African slaves and European planters. Creole is a composite of several languages: French, Indian, African, English and Spanish. Despite the higher status accorded to the speaking of French, Creole remains the popular language of Haitians and is spoken and/or understood by all classes (Cosgray, 1991; Romain, 1978). Translations of some Creole and French expressions are presented at the end of this chapter.

Haitian Americans often gesture with their hands as they speak. They are usually comfortable with direct eye contact and touch and frequently use both to indicate friendship during a conversation. These clients tend to react positively to direct eye contact, a touch, or a smile by the health professional (Cosgray, 1991).

SOCIOECONOMIC STATUS

The Haitian community, often referred to as *kominote*, is usually highly differentiated. The major divisions are the elite and the people or the masses (*pep-la* or *mas-la*). The elite are a minority of individuals who enjoy the highest social status by virtue of their wealth, intelligence, education, and political position. They usually speak French, as well as Creole, and frequently English also. *Pep-la* refers to the larger percentage of Haitians who are of lower social status, generally less educated, and speak only Creole (Buchanan, 1983). Similar to European immigrants in the United States, Haitian-American immigrants have developed their own unique subculture that is distinct from the mainstream American culture (Laguerre, 1984).

Some Haitian-American communities in New York are divided with respect to social class and color, legacies of their colonial slave-based past. *Klass* is the term that some Haitian Americans use to designate social categories on the basis of wealth, family name and ancestry, education, and color. These divisions constitute a social hierarchy brought from Haiti and reinstituted in the United States (Buchanan, 1983; Cosgray, 1991).

Although many factors associated with *klass* in Haiti are no longer important in the United States, ancestry or family name may persist in some communities as an important social class factor. Some families, referred to as the *gran fanmi* (great families) experience a long history of importance and prestige because of their political, economic, and intellectual accomplishments in Haiti. Prominent family names are often recognized throughout the Haitian-American community (Buchanan, 1983). Many middle-class immigrants were able to establish themselves in comparable professional fields, which placed them on the American middle-class level. However, without the proper credentials and the nepotism to which they were accustomed, some of the former bourgeoisie were forced to take menial jobs in America, whereas some of the lower-class immigrants, with marketable skills (e.g., as auto mechanics, carpenters) and new opportunities for education, were able to rise quickly on the socioeconomic ladder (Buchanan, 1983).

CHIEF COMPLAINT

Harwood (1981) observed that by the time some Haitian Americans consulted an American health professional, they tended to have already formed their own diagnosis. Some may tell the professional what disease they think they have rather than describe the symptoms. If the client's concept of disease is holistic (illness is related to the entire body), this individual might view the accurate description of localized pain as unimportant for diagnosis (Laguerre, 1984).

Illness may cause shame for some Haitian Americans. Serious illness is discussed only with family members and close friends. In Haitian culture, illness should be accepted heroically. Traditionally it has been believed that an individual must be strong because psychological weakness will allow the illness to dominate the body. Public displays of weakness are not condoned. Thus, placing a client in a wheelchair may indicate serious illness publicly displayed. This routine hospital practice may elicit negative emotions in some traditional Haitian-American clients (Laguerre, 1984).

FAMILY

The Haitian family is usually extended and patriarchal in Haiti and in America. Lower-class one-parent families tend to be matriarchal.

After becoming established in America, new immigrants are morally obligated to send for other family members, although it may take several years for an entire family to become reunited in the United States. This vast kinship network, spanning two countries, perpetuates the extended family system (Leavitt & Lutz, 1988). Haitian Americans generally maintain contact with family in Haiti by sending remittances or visiting on vacation or for special occasions, particularly during Carnival and for funerals. Sometimes children are sent to Haiti to be cared for by relatives and educated in Haitian schools. This practice frees Haitian-American parents to work and save toward the purchase of a home and at the same time provides a preferred education for the child that focuses on the French language, Christian principles, and Haitian customs (Laguerre, 1984).

The Haitian family is usually a closely knit, supportive group. In a study by Lassiter (1988), most Haitian informants described their families as strict, rigid, and protective. One informant added that there was "little touching and verbal expressions of affection among her family members." However, togetherness and communication were characteristics of most Haitian families. Similar to other ethnic groups, family behavior is a function of socioeconomic status or social class.

Settlement in the United States has had little or no effect on the sex roles of Haitian men and women. The home is frequently considered the Haitian woman's domain, and she has limited interest in community affairs, whereas the man's domain is outside the house (Leavitt & Lutz, 1988). Laguerre (1984) noted that some Haitian women in New York tended to be more assertive and independent than they were in Haiti. One factor responsible for this change may be her ability to achieve economic independence in America. Consequently, the gender roles in many Haitian-American families have tended to become less traditional and more egalitarian.

Laguerre (1984) identifies four types of marriages and household organizations:

1. *Mariag de goudin*. For the purpose of becoming eligible for resident status, a middle-class or upper-class Haitian living in the United States marries a lower-class individual who is a citizen or has a resident visa.

2. *Mariag residans*. Two Haitians of similar social status marry when only one has resident status.

3. *Mariag bay bous*. Marriage is contracted between a person with resident status and a person in Haiti, frequently arranged by the kin.

4. *Bon mariag*. Marriage is arranged for a couple, both of the same status, before they migrate to America or after residence, for the purpose of establishing a relationship and a family.

The first three unions are for purposes of immigration, to facilitate entry into the United States, the fourth type is the only one entered into for the purpose of forming a household. Another type of union, not legally recognized in the United States, is the consensual union; it generally has difficulty remaining intact after migration (Laguerre, 1984).

CHILD REARING

Usually both Haitian-American parents work, so day care must be provided for their children, usually by other Haitian women who live nearby. Haitian mothers prefer this arrangement because they find that community child care facilities have inflexible hours, do not offer personalized care, and are too expensive (Leavitt & Lutz, 1988).

Although Haitian parents are usually extremely loving and affectionate with their children, they are also strict and authoritarian. Child rearing may be shared by siblings as well as parents. Children are taught to show unquestioned obedience to their elders. Children do not usually ask their parents questions about intimate subjects such as sex because this would be disrespectful (Cosgray, 1991). Some parents tend to employ physical punishment, the same disciplinary method used by their parents in Haiti. Haitian-American parents generally do not like professional counseling and/or assignment to parenting groups. They feel that other individuals from diverse cultural groups view children's behavior from a different perspective. One way of dealing with a child whom parents feel they cannot control is to send the child to Haiti to live with kin (Fouron, 1983).

Some Haitian-American children face adaptation difficulties in the United States because they are torn between two cultures. Their peers encourage them to become Americanized, while their families try to maintain Haitian cultural traditions. Generally these children elect to speak English even at home, while their parents continue to speak Creole or French. Most American-born children have become socialized to mainstream American culture and, unlike their parents, have little interest in returning to Haiti. Some adult Haitian-American children who are successfully employed show little enthusiasm for contributing money to fulfill their parents' economic obligations in Haiti or to bring kin and friends to America. This practice sometimes causes intergenerational conflict (Fouron, 1983).

SOCIALIZATION PATTERNS

Some Haitian Americans who adhere to the principles of social class may attempt to perpetuate this traditional class system in the United States based on wealth, language, and color (Buchanan-Stafford, 1987). However, many other Haitian Americans believe that a good education and professionalism can elevate one's social class, regardless of ancestry. Comportment and proper behavior are important indicators of class. Proper behavior includes good manners, a modulated speaking voice, avoidance of public scenes, refraining from profanity, and appearing neat and clean at all times. Friends should be carefully selected, keeping in mind the expression, "Birds of a feather flock together." Improper behavior is considered an embarrassment to one's family and upbringing and may reflect on one's parents' ineffectiveness as disciplinary agents (Buchanan, 1983).

I interviewed 24 Haitian Americans in New York, asking them to describe their personality. Most described themselves as "a nice person"; no one offered a negative self-description, except for expressions of shyness. A larger percentage of the women (69%) than the men (38%) described themselves as "shy and quiet." On the other hand, more men (38%) than women (25%) indicated a need for solitude. Frequent statements were, "I like to be alone to think things over," "I seldom feel lonely," and "I enjoy being alone." I found the Haitian Americans more reluctant than other groups (e.g., West Indian Americans and African Americans) to participate in the interviews. Haitian-American men were more reluctant than the women. They appeared to be very private people who were not prone to reveal personal information to a stranger (Lassiter, 1988).

The result of psychological studies by Bordeleau and Kline (1986) indicated that projection was a frequent defense mechanism among Haitians. Delusions were often related to voodoo religious beliefs. It was also noted that aggression was seldom directed toward others, and hyperactivity was usually more noisy than destructive. It was further noted that Haitians rarely commit suicide.

RELIGIOUS BELIEFS AND PRACTICES

Similar to many other Caribbean cultures, some Haitian Americans recognize two religions. Catholicism is usually considered the religion of Haiti. In America, the Catholic church, with services now offered in French and Creole (since 1966), plays an important supportive role in Haitian-American communities. Some Haitian Americans affiliate with other Protestant denominations: Baptist, Episcopal, Seventh Day Adventist, or Pentecostal (Leavitt & Lutz, 1988).

Haiti's second religion is voodoo (*Voudou, Voudoun, Vudum*), based on a set of beliefs about spirits and/or gods and their natural relationship to humans and the universe. People who practice voodoo may be Christians. In their belief the religions can coexist; one is not replaced by the other (Metraux, 1972).

African in origin, voodoo is an informal religion, practiced by autonomous groups and manifested by ceremonial rituals. Groups of adherents perpetuate and preserve these practices under a priest (*ongan, houngan*) or priestess (*mambo*). There is no church, so gatherings usually occur at the home or sanctuary (*hunfo*) of the *ongan* or *mambo*. Here believers worship supernatural beings (*lwa, loas, mysteres, saints,* or *angels*).

The voodoo religion is based on the belief of practitioners, or *protégés* as they are called, that a human is composed of a material or physical body and an invisible spiritual or psyche energy force. This invisible spirit (similar to the concept of soul) gives life to matter. When this spirit withdraws permanently, death is said to occur. This spirit or soul that exists in each human is the energy that activates the mind for all thought processes and motivates behavior (Cosgray, 1991; Laguerre, 1980).

Believers in voodoo perceive life in the universe in terms of a hierarchy. God is on the primary level, and humans, God's first creation, are on the second level. Deities, Catholic saints, and *loa* or spirits that govern human affairs occupy the third level. The *loa* (spirits of the dead) and *protégés* (believers) exist in an intimate relationship of interdependence. *Protégés* acknowledge the *loa* in regular ceremonies during which food and offerings are presented. The *loa*, in return, protect their *protégés* from illness and misfortune. Thus humans and spirits coexist in the universe in symbiotic relationships (Cosgray, 1991; Deren, 1970).

Possession occurs when a human soul is displaced by a *loa*, with the possession described as the *loa* "riding" or "mounting" the human, who then goes into a trance. The person being mounted is usually a member of a group involved in a religious voodoo ceremony. Possession does not mean that the individual can communicate with the spirit; instead, the person is merely a vehicle through which the spirit can reveal itself. During this special ceremony led by *hougans* or *mambos*, or both, and enhanced by ritualistic songs and dances, possession is viewed as a highly positive experience. Therefore the possessed person is considered privileged (Cosgray, 1991; Deren, 1970; Laguerre, 1984).

Voodoo flourished in Haiti because it was flexible and adaptive to people living close to nature. There was no need to keep records, because voodoo rituals, songs, and stories were passed down from generation to generation by elders through word of mouth. Certain symbols are drawn and known to represent particular spirits. Thus, Voodoo encompasses a set of unwritten beliefs and unique practices dealing with the spiritual forces of the universe for the purpose of helping individuals interact more effectively with their environments (Cosgray, 1991; Leyburn, 1966).

Although some Haitian Americans may practice voodoo (Cosgray, 1991), it is impossible to ascertain the number of practitioners in the United States for at least two reasons. First, many Haitian Americans from the middle and upper classes are generally unfamiliar with voodoo. Second, Haitian Americans who are believers are reluctant to admit it because of the stigma attached to voodoo.

CULTURALLY BASED HEALTH BELIEFS AND PRACTICES

The central Haitian folk concept of illness is that disease is a disruption of the balanced state of the blood. Traditionally various types of internal and external disruptions have been identified. For example, fright (*sezisman* in Creole, *saisissement* in French) is a system disruption caused by shock such as bad news or a threat to well-being. It is believed that *sezisman* causes blood to rush to the head, resulting in partial blindness, headaches, and temporary mental illness. It is thought that lactating mothers are particularly susceptible to this phenomenon (Laguerre, 1983).

A group of Haitian Americans in Miami reported a number of activities that they considered important for maintaining health: eating well, keeping regular hours, exercising regularly, and maintaining proper personal hygiene. Some cited prayer and good spiritual habits. Since Haitians Americans often relate food to health, many believe that fat people are healthier and happier than thin people (Laguerre, 1984).

Similar to many people from other traditional cultures, some Haitian Americans tend to manifest an external locus of control. Thus, they may perceive disease as caused by factors external to the body, such as "cold" or "hot" air or foods, "gas," and spirits. But many of these individuals, especially those of lower economic status, have great difficulty accepting the theory that a germ (also an external factor) can cause disease. This external locus of control often prevents introspection, which may avert attempts to assume control of one's body. Therefore, disease prevention and therapeutic measures such as relaxation training and biofeedback could be ineffective with these clients (Laguerre, 1984).

Some Haitian Americans perceive disease as divided into two broad categories: natural illness and supernatural illness. Natural illnesses are those with familiar symptoms and are generally of short duration. The most dangerous types of illness are believed to be caused by irregularities in the blood, which include the following:

- *San cho* ("hot" blood) provokes a high fever. Blood becomes "hot" when one is nervous or involved in intellectual activities and during physical activity or sleep. A woman's body is believed to be "hot" during the postpartum period, and diet is given to balance this state. The blood is said to be cold as a result of malaria or when the body is quiet and at rest.
- *San cle* (thin blood) causes pallor. The blood becomes thick in the case of fright or in hypertension.
- *San febel* (weak blood) causes physical or mental weakness.
- *San jo-n* (yellow blood) indicates the presence of bile in the blood.
- *San noa* (dark blood) indicates terminal illness (Harwood, 1981; Laguerre, 1984).

Gaz (gas) causes pain and anemia. Gas may enter the body through the ears, causing headaches, or through the mouth, causing stomachaches. It may move to other parts of the body and cause pain in the back, shoulders, and/or extremities. Avoidance of leftover foods is thought to prevent gas.

Some believe that illness is caused by an imbalance of hot and cold elements, especially in foods. Foods are classified as hot or cold. Therefore, a food or medicine of the opposite category would be used to treat a person in a cold-hot system (Harwood, 1981; Leavitt & Lutz, 1988).

Diseases of supernatural origin are believed to be caused by angry spirits. Spirits and believers (*protégés*) are interdependent. Ceremonies are held periodically to honor one's spirits, which in turn provide protection. Some believe that disease may occur if the *protégé* fails to honor the spirits properly and periodically, and illness becomes the punishment. Voodoo priests are the primary sources for diagnosis and treatment of supernatural diseases. Thus voodoo is both a religion and a therapeutic system (Cosgray, 1991; Laguerre, 1984).

Traditionally it has been believed that since the postpartum period is the most crucial period for the mother, she must keep warm, drink special teas, and take warm baths containing therapeutic leaves. These activities are considered essential for cleansing and restoration of her natural state. In addition, at about one month postpartum, some believe that she must take a cold bath followed by self-induced vomiting in order to complete the cleansing process (Jeanty, 1989). Some Haitian Americans may believe that the postpartum woman is susceptible to the entrance of gas after birth, so after delivery, she is encouraged to wear a tight belt around her waist to prevent the gas from entering her body. Gas can be treated with a special tea made from garlic, mint, and cloves or by eating such solid foods as plantain and corn. The hot tea and foods classed as "heavy" stimulate the intestinal tract to expel gas (Snow, 1985).

Traditionally it has also been believed that the milk of a nursing mother can be displaced or spoiled by the mother's emotions. Consequently, family and friends try not to provoke a lactating mother into losing her temper, because this could result in harm to herself and her baby. Some believe that milk may rise to the mother's brain and cause acute headache, postpartum depression, and/or psychoses. Also, the possible danger exists that if the milk mixes with the mother's blood it could poison the nursing baby (Snow, 1985).

Another traditional belief is that of the wandering womb, a displaced womb or uterus, which is believed to occur during the early postpartum period. Because the womb and the baby are said to have established a strong relationship during gestation, it is thought that the deserted womb after birth may wander around the body in search of its lost occupant. This wandering womb may travel into any part of the mother's body. Symptoms such as weakness, dizziness, and confusion, which are experienced by many women during the postpartum period, are believed to be caused by this displaced womb that is wandering around looking for its lost inhabitant. Traditionally, in rural Haiti, a skilled midwife would perform a series of massages to return the uterus to its proper place (Snow, 1985).

Perdition is another traditional belief found among some Haitian Americans. Perdition is a condition in which a woman has a fetus trapped in her uterus possibly for several years, before finally giving birth to the baby. Perdition is thought to originate from practices such as walking barefoot on wet surfaces or lifting heavy objects. In perdition, the development of the fetus is arrested and the growth process reversed during early pregnancy. The fetus then returns to its original size, a microscopic speck, and remains in this state for several months or years. Although she may menstruate, the woman is believed to remain in perdition until the pregnancy becomes obvious. When the problem that provoked the perdition no longer exists, the fetus begins to grow and develop normally, to be born after nine months with no untoward effects. The concept of perdition in traditional Haitian culture may have served several purposes. It reduced the stigma of infertility because a woman in perdition was not considered sterile; her pregnancy was merely on hold. Since sterility was grounds for dissolving a conjugal union, perdition could have secured a union. Furthermore, a woman in perdition was regarded as having a higher status than a nonpregnant woman (Snow, 1985).

Laguerre (1984) noted that some Haitian Americans seek treatment for illness generally in the following sequence: home remedies, modern medicine, folk healers, voodoo medicine, or a return trip to Haiti to visit a special healer or doctor. Although many Haitian Americans tend to try home remedies first and then perhaps a healer, they usually consult a mainstream health professional early for illness in their children. Generally, reasons for a delay in going to a mainstream health provider are varied and may include insufficient finances for private care, not wanting to lose a day from work to attend a clinic, or fear of revealing undocumented status. Pain and weakness are the motivating symptoms that will cause the Haitian individual to seek this care, they like a thorough examination including expert use of the stethoscope, few questions, a quick diagnosis, and perhaps an injection or a prescription (Harwood, 1981).

CULTURAL DIETARY PATTERNS

The Haitian-American community maintains many of its cultural dietary traditions through local food stores, bakeries, and restaurants that supply favorite Haitian foodstuffs. Haitian music is frequently enjoyed by the family while eating the evening meal. Due to work schedules in America, the main meal is often the evening meal. In Haiti the heavy main meal is usually enjoyed around midday, followed by a light evening supper (Laguerre, 1984).

A typical meal of a middle-class Haitian-American family is similar to that of other Caribbean families. The meal might consist of a peas and rice mixture, fried plantains, corn, a meat (chicken, beef, pork, or goat) marinated in a spicy creole sauce, avocado, and orange or papaya juice. Haitian food is usually highly seasoned (Laguerre, 1984). Harwood (1981) noted that Haitian-American clients have difficulty maintaining therapeutic dietary restrictions, which can pose serious concerns in the treatment of diabetes, cardiovascular disorders, and gastric ulcers.

Favorite Haitian-American foods are rice, beef, goat meat, chicken, fish, okra, sweet potatoes, pumpkin, sugar cane, breadfruit, plantains, kidney beans, biscuits, and cassava bread. Favorite fruits and nuts are avocados, cashew nuts, coconuts, mangoes, bananas, grapefruit, limes, pineapples, and star apples (Cosgray, 1991).

Some Haitian Americans classify foods in terms of hot and cold, unrelated to temperature. Some foods that are considered very cold are avocado, coconut, and mango. Examples of cool foods are orange juice, cane syrup, and tomato. Coffee, nutmeg, and rum exemplify very hot foods, and eggs and grapefruit juice are classified as warm foods. Several foods are considered neutral, neither hot nor cold: breadfruit, cabbage, coconut candy, fish, goat meat, pigeon peas, plantain, white and brown rice, and kidney beans (Harwood, 1981; Laguerre, 1984).

MORBIDITY AND MORTALITY

Between November 1991 and April 1992, approximately 18,000 Haitian migrants received medical care and medical screening required for entry into the United States. The most common diseases found were:

Fever/malaria, 35%

Otis media, URI, 10%

Measles, 6%

Pneumonia, 4%

Varicella, 4%

Cellulitis, 2%

Filariasis, 2%

Malaria was the most common disease noted among Haitian immigrants.

As required by the Immigration Act of 1990, the medical staff performed tests for syphilis, HIV, and tuberculosis on the migrants and found the following percentages (Morbidity and Mortality Weekly Report, 1993):

Syphilis, 5%

HIV positive, 7%

TB, 5%

Because of unproved statements about AIDS in Haiti, some sources in the United States promoted a fear and stigma about AIDS in the Haitian population and prevented Haitians from donating blood. This stigma is decreasing (Laverdiere, Tremblay, Lavallee, Bonny, Lacome & Boileau, 1983). Health professionals should keep in mind that Haitians are no longer classified as a high-risk group by the Centers for Disease Control (Fain, 1984).

BELIEFS ABOUT DEATH AND DYING

Haitian Americans who practice voodoo believe in the symbiotic existence of humans and spirits of the dead. Some believe that if the child's soul is captured and placed in a bottle, that person will live until that bottle is broken. Some believe that zombies are doomed to live after death because they were cursed by an enemy. If one strongly believes this, one might request that after death his or her body parts be buried in separate graves to avoid becoming a zombie (Cosgray, 1991). Haitians who adhere solely to Catholicism endorse beliefs about death and dying in keeping with the doctrines of the Catholic church.

PHYSICAL ASSESSMENT

Haitians are of African origin and are similar physically and biologically to African Americans. Skin tones range from fair to dark brown. See the physical assessment section in Chapter 1 on African Americans.

Translations of Some Common Haitian Terms

English	Creole
I do not feel well.	*Kom pa bon.*

I am convalescing.	*Moin an konvalesans.*
I am sick.	*Moin malad.*
I am very sick.	*Moin malad anpil.*
Hypertension	*Tension*
Quick diagnosis	*Rapidité de diagnostique*

English	**French**
Hello, good day	*Bonjour*
How are you?	*Comment allez-vous?*
Yes	*Oui*
No	*Non*
Nurse	*Infirmiere*
Doctor	*Docteur*
Thank you	*Merci*
Minister	*Pasteur*
Priest	*Prêtre*
Husband	*Mari*
Wife	*Epouse*
Mother	*Mère*
Father	*Père*
Social worker	*Assistante sociale*
Psychologist	*Psychologue*
Pain	*Douleur*
Hot	*Chaud*
Cold	*Froid*
Numb	*Engourdi*
Hungry	*Faim*
Thirsty	*Soif*
Short of breath	*Essoufflé*
Allergic	*Allergie*
Food	*Nourriture*
Medicine	*Médecine*
Urinal	*Urinoir*
Bedpan	*Bassin*
Bath	*Bain*
Oxygen	*Oxygene*
Blanket	*Cauverture*

Water	*Eau*
Coffee	*Café*
Tissues	*Mouchoirs cellulose*
Dentures	*Dentiers*
Money	*Argent*
Leave me alone.	*Laissez moi seul.*
No visitors	*Pas de visiteurs*
Get out of bed.	*Levez-vous.*
Back to bed	*Au lit*
Sit down	*Asseyez-vous*
Walk	*Marchez*
Go home	*A la maison*
TV	*TV*
Radio	*Radio*
On	*Allumer*
Off	*Eteindre*
Change	*Changer*
Goodbye	*Adieu, au revoir*

Sources: Creole/English from Harwood, 1981; Laguerre, 1983. French/English from Beamatic Communicator. Courtesy of Omnimed Inc., Pine Avenue, P.O. Box 446, Maple Shade, NJ 08052-0446.

REFERENCES

Bordeleau, J. M., & Kline, N. S. (1986). Experience in developing psychiatric services in Haiti. *World Mental Health*, pp. 170–83.

Buchanan, S. H. (1983). The cultural meaning of class for Haitians in New York City. *Ethnic Groups, 5* (1&2), 7–29.

Buchanan-Stafford, S. (1987). Language and identity: Haitians in New York City. In C. R. Sutton & E. M. Chaney (Eds.), *Caribbean life in New York City: Sociocultural dimensions* (pp. 202–17). Staten Island, NY: Center for Migration Studies of New York.

Bureau of the Census. (1992). *Statistical abstract of the United States*. Washington, DC: Government Printing Office.

Chaney, E. M. (1987). The context of Caribbean migration. In C. Sutton & E. Chaney (Eds.), *Caribbean life in New York City: Sociocultural dimensions* (pp. 3–14). Staten Island, NY: Center for Migration Studies of New York.

Cosgray, R. E. (1991). Haitian Americans. In J. N. Giger & R. E. Davidhizar (Eds.), *Transcultural nursing: Assessment and intervention* (pp. 465–88). St. Louis: Mosby Year Book.

Deren, M. (1970). *Divine horseman: Voodoo Gods of Haiti*. New York: Chelsea House Publishers.

Fain, N. (1984, September 18). Health. *Advocate*, 6–9.

Fouron, G. (1983). The black dilemma in the U.S.: The Haitian experience. *Journal of Caribbean Studies, 3*(3), 242–65.

Harwood, A. (1981). *Ethnicity and medical care*. Cambridge: Harvard University Press.

Jeanty, M. (1989). Personal communication.

Laguerre, M. S. (1980). *Voodoo heritage*. Beverly Hills: Sage Publications.

Laguerre, M. S. (1984). *American odyssey: Haitians in New York City*. Ithaca: Cornell University Press.

Lassiter, S. M. (1988). *Coping as a function of culture and socio-economic status for Haitians and Africans*. Unpublished study, Adelphi University, New York.

Laverdiere, M., Tremblay, J., Lavallee, R., Bonny, Y., Lacombe, M., & Boileau, J. (1983). AIDS in Haitian immigrants and in a Caucasian woman closely associated with Haitians. *Canadian Medical Association Journal, 129*(11), 1209–12.

Leavitt R., & Lutz, M. E. (1988). *Three immigrant groups in New York City: Dominicans, Haitians, and Cambodians*. New York: Community Council of Greater New York.

Leyburn, J. G. (1966). *The Haitian people*. New Haven: Yale University Press.

Metraux, G. (1972). *Voodoo in Haiti*. New York: Schocken Books.

Morbidity and Mortality Weekly Report. (1993). *Health status of Haitian migrants: U.S. Naval Base, Guantanamo Bay, Cuba, November 1991–April 1992*, pp. 138–140. U.S. Department of Health and Human Services/Public Health Services/CDC.

Romain, J. B. (1978). Cultural values: Identification, dangers, lines of action. *Cultures, 5*(3), 90–109.

Schiller, N. G., DeWind, J., Brutus, M. L., Charles, C., Fouron, F., & Thomas, A. (1987). All in the same boat? Unity and diversity in Haitian organizing in New York. In C. R. Sutton & E. M. Chaney (Eds.), *Caribbean life in New York City: Sociocultural dimensions* (pp. 182–201). Staten Island, NY: Center for Migration Studies of New York.

Snow, J. Public Health Group. (1985). *Common health care beliefs and practices of Puerto Ricans, Haitians and low income Black living in New York/New Jersey area*. NHSC/DHHS Region 11, Contract 120-83-0011.

9

Irish Americans

The Republic of Ireland, located in northwestern Europe, covers approximately 85% of the island that bears its name. It consists of 26 counties that became the Irish Free State in 1921. The country is called Eire, the Emerald Isle, because of its beautiful green countryside.

The Republic of Ireland is bordered on the northeast by Northern Ireland and on the west and south by the Atlantic Ocean. The St. George's Channel, the Irish Sea, and the North Channel separate Ireland from the United Kingdom, about 50 miles distant. Ireland's climate is cool and damp. In summer temperatures range from about 57 to 61 degrees F. The winters are mild, with temperatures averaging between 40 and 44 degrees F (Martin, 1991).

POPULATION IN THE UNITED STATES

About 15.6% of the American population—about 38.5 million people—are of Irish descent. The Irish are the second leading foreign-born ancestry group in the United States (Germans are first, and the English are third). The largest Irish population resides in the South (33%), followed by the Midwest (25%), Northeast (24%), and West (15%). Large numbers of Irish live in North and South Carolina, Alabama, Louisiana, Texas, and New York (Bureau of the Census, 1992).

Immigrants who arrived in America in the 1700s were predominantly Protestant, mainly Presbyterian from northwestern Ireland (Ulster). The Protestant Irish were often called the Scots-Irish to differentiate them from the Catholic Irish.

COMMUNICATION

Ireland has two official languages, English, spoken with an accent known as a brogue, and Gaelic, usually called Irish (Martin, 1991).

Some Irish prefer a wide personal space zone. Some actually have more difficulty expressing feelings to close family members than to distant persons (Greeley, 1981; Martin, 1991). Many Irish individuals have a keen respect for personal boundaries and are sensitive to individual rights to privacy (McGoldrick, 1982).

SOCIOECONOMIC STATUS

Many early immigrants, former farmers in Ireland, worked as unskilled laborers in America on the railroads and in factories. White-collar Irish were most often employed as teachers, clergy, or politicians. Irish Americans have been highly represented in the police and fire departments (Daniels, 1990). In 1960, Senator John F. Kennedy became the first Irish Roman Catholic elected president of the United States.

CHIEF COMPLAINT

Irish clients are most likely to locate problems in the eyes, ears, nose, and throat. This may be a symbolic representation of the source, sin and guilt. For example, these areas of focus may reflect beliefs as to what should have been seen, heard, or said (Martin, 1991).

Irish clients sometimes deny that pain is a part of their illness or describe pain as more of a throbbing or pinprick than actual pain. The philosophy of guilt and sin promotes the belief that pain and suffering are inevitable to be experienced in silence since they are punishment for sins. Some Irish individuals view suffering as deserved because of personal guilt. Irish individuals appear to have a much higher tolerance for physical pain than persons of many other cultural groups. They tend to be noncomplaining, silent sufferers, often even in the presence of family members, and may not seek relief until the pain becomes extremely severe, and even then they may tend to understate their physical discomfort (Martin, 1991; McGoldrick, 1982).

FAMILY

The family system places its welfare above that of each individual, with the father accepting the responsibility for the economic welfare of the family members and children accepting differential treatment in the interest of the total family (Horgan, 1988).

The family of the nineteenth century was a modified, bilateral, extended kinship system that stressed male dominance and blood and sibling loyalty. The father designated a son, usually the eldest, as inheritor of the family property. When this son or heir married, the bride presented a dowry not to her husband but to his father, in an amount equal to the value of the father's property. The couple then moved in with the son's parents, a situation sometimes causing tensions between the new bride and the mother-in-law. If a father had no sons, a daughter became the heiress, and when she married, the groom presented her father with a significant amount of money. The father often made provisions for other children of the family with the money obtained from a dowry.

Traditionally women have been subservient to the men of the family, and male needs have been prioritized. A notably high number of single women among the Irish immigrants may have promoted early manifestations of feminism (Horgan, 1988). But although they are considered subservient, Irish women are often viewed as morally superior to men because they are conceptualized as a reflection of the Virgin Mary. They are often seen as independent and dominant (Kennedy, 1978). When compared to other Anglo-American women, Irish women have been found to perceive their role of wife-mother as the dominant one in marriage. Careers have been less important (Martin, 1991).

Delayed marriage was common among early Irish immigrants. The average marriage age for women was 31, and the typical age for men was 35 (Horgan, 1988).

Traditional Irish families are characterized by favoritism toward sons, attitude of male authority, families obliged to care for one another, sibling loyalty, limited amount of overt affection, heavy use of alcohol to increase sociability, and residence in parishes, with the Catholic church at the center of the community.

The modern American Catholic Irish family is patriarchal and nuclear in structure, with the father as the head. Typical ages at marriage are 22 for women and 24.5 for men—somewhat earlier than for early Irish immigrants. Although women tend to view their family as more important than a career, enthusiasm for feminism has increased. Parents now exercise less authority over the marriages of their children.

Abortion and homosexuality are viewed with disfavor, and divorce and extramarital affairs are not common (Horgan, 1988; Martin, 1991).

ELDERLY

Some children prefer to extend their family to include the elderly; others prefer to use private or public care facilities. Thus, American Catholic Irish families demonstrate diverse behaviors with respect to the care of older adults (Horgan, 1988).

CHILD REARING

Traditionally, the Irish Catholic mother has been firm and highly moralistic but also kind and sentimental. Discipline is often maintained through ridicule, mocking, belittling, and/or shaming. In families where alcohol is abused, discipline may be inappropriate and harsh (Martin, 1991).

Children are taught to be subordinate, polite, obedient, and respectful. A study that compared Irish and Italians (Vosburgh & Juliani, 1990) found that good manners and obedience to parents were rated more important by Italians and other whites than by the Irish. Instead, the values of self-control, curiosity, and independence were stressed more by Irish individuals.

Boys may be treated with more affection than girls by their mothers. Fathers teach boys how to fight (an honorable skill) in order to stand up for their rights. Children's success may be sometimes underplayed and taken for granted. Traditionally, sexual expression is discouraged (McGoldrick, 1982). A number of Irish Catholic children attend parochial schools that emphasize discipline and reinforce their Irish culture (McGoldrick, 1982).

SOCIALIZATION PATTERNS

The Irish culture places a high value on conformity and respectability, yet some individuals tend toward eccentricity. The Irish emphasize loyalty to their own, but they often sever relationships completely.

Some Irish have been described as sexually repressed. It is believed that some may avoid tenderness and affection; emotions are kept under control by guilt feelings (McGoldrick, 1982; Martin, 1991). Repression of sexual expression, body attitudes, and intimate contact may be exemplified by the traditional dance, the Irish jig. When doing the jig, skilled dancers move only their feet while keeping the rest of the body as motionless and inexpressive as possible (McGoldrick, 1982).

Many Irish are highly articulate, with an affinity for verbal innuendos. Many turn to dreams and fantasy when frustrated, and so poets are valued members of the Irish society (Martin, 1991). Yet many Irish may demonstrate an inability to express inner feelings. This characteristic presents serious problems for counselors and therapists (McGoldrick, 1982).

RELIGIOUS BELIEFS AND PRACTICES

Most Irish people are Roman Catholic; others are Protestant, particularly Presbyterian and Methodist. The Irish are active managers in the church, and a large percentage of priests and bishops are of Irish ancestry (Horgan, 1988). St. Patrick, one of the early missionaries during the eighth century, established a strong church in Ireland, which spread through continental Europe. The Catholic church has continued to maintain a strong following in America (McGoldrick, 1982). Marriage is preferably to another Irish person or at least to another Catholic. A non-Catholic marriage partner is urged to convert and to raise the children in the Catholic faith (Horgan, 1988).

The Catholic religion is the basis for the Irish strong sense of sin and guilt.

An underlying belief is that people are essentially bad and deserve to suffer for their sins. This philosophy is related to original sin: in spite of all efforts, one cannot escape human nature, which is basically evil and prone to sin.

Catholic philosophy holds that all sins committed in one's lifetime must be suffered after death in purgatory before the soul can go to heaven. Mortal sins prevent one's soul from going to purgatory or heaven after death. Mortal sins include murder, lying, theft, disobedience to parents and other authority figures, sinful thoughts, use of contraceptives, adultery, abortion, divorce, and suicide (Horgan, 1988). Periodic confessions to a priest are required to absolve sin and free one's soul. This is particularly important for the dying client. Irish-Catholic babies are baptized by a priest, at which time they receive a saint's name. Godparents, selected at this time, are responsible for seeing that the child remains a Catholic until marriage. Many Irish Americans manifest an external locus of control based on the Catholic belief of original sin (Horgan, 1988; Martin, 1991).

CULTURALLY BASED HEALTH BELIEFS AND PRACTICES

Some Irish Americans perceive illness as a self-fulfilling prophesy related to the concept of sin and guilt (Martin, 1991). Folk practices include the following:

- Blessing of the throat.
- Wearing holy medals will prevent illness.
- Wearing a bag cf camphor around the neck will prevent the flu.
- Onions under the bed keep nasal passages clear.
- Never go to bed with wet hair.
- Eat lots of oily foods.
- Maintain a strong, loving family to prevent illness.
- Cleanse the bowels once a week with senna.
- Eat a balanced diet, and take vitamins to stay healthy.
- Think positively along with exercise and adequate rest to foster optimal wellness.
- Nurture strong religious beliefs to promote good health.
- See a doctor only in an emergency (Martin, 1991; Spector, 1991).

Individuals of Irish descent do not usually ascribe to special folk healers. However, members of the family (especially older women) may serve as health consultants, forming a lay referral system (Chrisman & Kleinman, 1980).

CULTURAL DIETARY PATTERNS

Irish cooking is simple. Principal foods include lamb, beef, pork, fruit, and potatoes. For many years potatoes have been a favorite food in the Irish diet. Boiled potatoes and potato pancakes are popular. One of Ireland's favorite traditional dishes is Irish stew, made by boiling potatoes, onions, and mutton in a covered pot. Another traditional dish consists of boiled salt pork, cabbage, and potatoes. Beer is the favorite alcoholic drink in Ireland. Irish whiskey made with barley malt is a famous liquor. Irish coffee, another favorite, is made with coffee, Irish whiskey, brown sugar, and cream.

In preparation for Holy Communion in the morning, an individual will begin fasting at midnight (Horgan, 1988). A notable dietary law in the past was the Roman Catholic ban on eating meat on Friday. However this ban was lifted during the reign of Pope John XXIII (Ensminger, Ensminger, Konlande & Robson, 1983).

MORBIDITY AND MORTALITY

The Irish tend to have a high incidence of alcoholism. Among American ethnic groups, Irish Americans have been ranked as one of the highest in terms of heavy alcohol intake and loss of control (Department of Health, Education and Welfare, 1971; Estes & Heinemann, 1986; Walsh & Walsh, 1973).

Northern Ireland has the highest incidence of coronary heart disease in the world (Riddoch, Savage, Murphy, Cran & Boreham, 1991).

Irish women in Ireland appear to be particularly vulnerable to ischemic heart disease and certain types of cancer. In comparison to several other European countries, Irish standardized mortality rates were the highest for women dying from lung cancer. The Irish standardized mortality rates were the highest for nonrheumatic heart diseases and respiratory tuberculosis for urban men and women, when compared to those for several other European countries. Some Irish women tend not to reveal symptoms related to poor health (Cook, 1990).

BELIEFS ABOUT DEATH AND DYING

For some American Catholic Irish, death is celebrated and seen as a welcome release from suffering. Therefore the wake is a prominent social event. (McGoldrick, 1982).

After preparation by a funeral parlor, the body is usually waked at home for two days and two nights. The casket remains open. A rosary is entwined between the fingers of the deceased. Friends and relatives who attend may offer contributions to the church for a mass in memory of the deceased. The women usually stay in the parlor with the casket, while the men congregate in the kitchen. Talk is generally of happy or humorous events related to the deceased, with much reminiscing. After the wake, the funeral parlor transports the deceased and the family to the church for the funeral mass. Burial follows, usually at a Catholic cemetery, after which a luncheon is held at the family home. Cremation is generally taboo (Horgan, 1988).

REFERENCES

Blessing, P. J. (1980). Irish. In S. Thernstrom (Ed.), *Harvard encyclopedia of American ethnic groups* (pp. 524–45). Cambridge: Belknap Press of Harvard University Press.

Bureau of the Census. (1992). *Statistical abstract of the United States.* Washington, DC: Government Printing Office.

Chrisman, N. J., & Kleinman, A. (1980). Health beliefs and practices. In S. Thernstrom (Ed.), *Harvard encyclopedia of American ethnic groups* (pp. 452–61) Cambridge: Belknap Press of Harvard university Press.

Cook, G. (1990). Health and social inequities in Ireland. *Social Science Medicine, 31*(3), 285–90.

Daniels, R. (1990). *Coming to America: A history of immigration and ethnicity in American life.* Princeton, NJ: HarperCollins.

Department of Health, Education and Welfare. (1971). *First special report to U.S. Congress on alcohol and health.* Washington, DC: Health Services and Mental Health Authority.

Ensminger, A. H., Ensminger, M. E., Konlande, J. E., & Robson, R. K. (1983). Religions and diets. In *Foods and nutrition encyclopedia* (Vol. 2), (pp. 1914–20). Clovis, CA: Pegus Press.

Estes, N., & Heinemann, M. E. (1986). *Alcoholism.* St. Louis: C. V. Mosby.

Greeley, A. (1981). *The Irish Americans.* New York: Harper & Row.

Horgan, E. S. (1988). The American Catholic Irish family. In C. H. Mindel, R. W. Haberstein, & R. Wright, Jr. (Eds.) *Ethnic families in America: Patterns and variations* (3d ed.) (pp. 45–75). New York: Elsevier.

Kennedy, R. E. (1978). *The Irish: Marriage, immigration and fertility.* Berkeley: University of California Press.

McGoldrick, M. (1982). Irish families. In M. McGoldrick, J. K. Pearce, & J. Giordano (Eds.), *Ethnicity and family therapy* (pp. 310–39). New York: Guilford Press.

Martin, C. (1991). Irish Americans. In J. N. Giger & R. E. Davidhizar (Eds.), *Transcultural nursing: Assessment and intervention* (pp. 315–33). New York: Mosby Year Book.

Riddoch, C., Savage, J. M., Murphy, N., Cran, G. W., & Boreham, C. (1991). Long term health implications of fitness and physical activity patterns. *Archives of Disease in Childhood, 66*(2), 1426–33.

Spector, R. (1991). *Cultural diversity in health and illness* (3d ed.). Norwalk, CT: Appleton & Lange.

Vosburgh, M. G., & Juliani, R. N. (1990). Contrasts in ethnic family patterns: The Irish and the Italians. *Journal of Comparative Family Studies, 21*(2), 269–86.

Walsh, B. M., & Walsh, D. (1973). Validity of indices of alcoholism: A comment from Irish experience. *British Journal of Preventive Social Medicine, 27*, 18–26.

10

Italian Americans

The Republic of Italy is located in southern Europe. The major part of Italy is a boot-shaped peninsula that projects in a direction from northwest to southeast into the Mediterranean Sea. Sicily and Sardinia, along with a number of small islands that are also part of Italy, lie to the west of the boot. Sicily, the largest island in the Mediterranean Sea, is located at the toe of the boot and is separated from the peninsula by the Strait of Messina. The island of Sardinia lies to the northwest, next to Corsica, which is part of France. Other small islands of Italy are Elba, Ischia, Capri, Giglio, Capraia, and the Lipari Islands.

Geographically, Italy is divided into the continental region in the north and the Mediterranean peninsula and insular regions in the south. The southern region is referred to as the Mezzogiorno. The climate of Italy varies by region. The mountains define the cold weather in the winter, especially in the north. The typical Mediterranean climate prevails in the southern peninsula and the islands. This is characterized by hot, dry summers and moderate winters with heavy annual rainfall (Bowen, 1991; Masur, 1985).

POPULATION IN THE UNITED STATES

Italians number about 14 million, or 5.9% of the American population. The largest number of Italian Americans reside in the Northeast (51%), with smaller numbers in the Midwest (17%), the South (17%), and the West (15%). Although most early Italian immigrants settled in San Francisco during the gold rush, today the largest population are found in New York, followed by Maine and Connecticut (Bureau of the Census, 1992).

COMMUNICATION

Italian is the language of Italy. Translations of some common Italian terms are listed at the end of this chapter.

Italians tend to express more emotional tension and stress than many other cultural groups. Sometimes their communication is characterized by loud-pitched voices with much gesturing and a dramatic expression of feelings (Rotunno & McGoldrick, 1982). Generally individuals of Italian descent prefer a close personal space, about 18 inches to 2 feet. Touching is usually acceptable, and a firm handshake is appropriate (Giger & Davidhizar, 1991; Watson, 1970). It is likely that the Italian American will prefer direct eye contact during communication (Bowen, 1991; Watson, 1970).

Italian Americans may be reluctant to trust outsiders, especially with personal information. If an interpreter is required, the client is likely to be more expressive if a family member, rather than a stranger, serves in this capacity.

SOCIOECONOMIC STATUS

A majority of Italian Americans trace their ancestry to the southern regions of Italy, the Mezzogiorno. The southern Italians developed different customs, life-styles and food preferences from northern Italians. Due to industrialization, Italians of the northern cities progressed financially and were able to lead relatively prosperous lives. The southern Italians, referred to as the *contadini*, meaning peasants or townspeople, were mainly farmers, less educated and poorer, and migrated more frequently to other parts of Europe, Africa, and the United States, seeking economic improvement.

Early Italian-American occupations were mainly manual labor. Some of these migrants obtained their jobs through ethnic labor contractors, the *padrone*; wages were low and living conditions in crowded tenements were grim.

Because of strong family attachments and a disdain for socializing with *stanieri* (outsiders), Italian Americans organized fewer communal groups and were less interested in education than other immigrant groups (Squier & Quadagno, 1988). In addition, disinterest in education (especially by the *contadini*), was fostered by an old Sicilian proverb: "Do not make your children better than yourself" (Ianni & Reuss-Ianni, 1972).

Despite the delay in gaining education, many Italian-American families have established and maintained income levels above the national average (Bureau of the Census, 1980). Some Italians in California established vineyards and became successful winemakers, and others became famous in politics, literature, and the arts (Daniels, 1990). Fiorello H. La Guardia was elected to Congress in 1916 and in the 1930s became a recognized leader as mayor of New York City. Today, Italian Mario Cuomo, former governor of New York State, is recognized nationally.

CHIEF COMPLAINT

Italian-American clients may describe symptoms dramatically with great detail, accompanied by gestures, facial expressions, and emotional intonations (Bowen, 1991).

FAMILY

The extended family was the norm in southern Italy, but the nuclear family is more common in northern Italy and in the United States. Kin generally live in close proximity, especially those of lower socioeconomic levels. A large network of significant others includes aunts, uncles, cousins, *gumbares* (old friends and neighbors), and godparents, who are also important in child rearing. Kin or relatives outside the household are expected to be more compliant and trustworthy than unrelated people, and kin are relied on for favors, loans, advice, socializing, and cooperative work. The proximity of residence often determines the importance of the kin.

The traditional father maintains an authoritative and distant stance, expecting obedience and respect from family members. Often a family council headed by the *capo di famiglio*, usually the father, makes decisions on a child's education, a cousin's dowry, a daughter's wedding, or an aunt's funeral expenses (Squier & Quadagno, 1988).

The traditional father is the undisputed authoritative head of the family. Although the mother is indulgent and viewed as inferior to the father, she has a tremendous sense of power manifested by her influence on her children. Because the traditional father's work often kept him away a great deal of the time, the mother would develop a strong relationship with her children. Sometimes the relationship of a mother and son is strong enough to create later conflicts with a son's wife and family (Rotunno & McGoldrick, 1982).

Traditionally, there has been a clear distinction between males and females in social relationships, patterns of education, work force participation, and expected family roles. Wives have generally kept close to home, limiting exposure to strangers and preventing temptation. At home a wife and mother has enjoyed emotional domination over her children and a notable informal power, in contrast to her formal subordination to her husband and other men (Squier & Quadagno, 1988). Often mutual support and complementarity of the roles of husband and wife have taken precedence over intimacy in Italian marriages (Arenson, 1979). However, recent generations have displayed increasing egalitarianism of male-female roles, especially among Italian Americans of the higher socioeconomic levels (Bowen, 1990; Squier & Quadagno, 1988).

The strength of the Italian family promotes solidarity and reinforcement in times of stress. Italian-American families are among the most stable in the United States today, having a low rate of divorce and a low rate of single-parent households (Rotunno & McGoldrick, 1982).

ELDERLY

Italians treat their elderly with great respect and are extremely reluctant to admit older relatives to nursing homes (Cacciola, 1982; Ragucci, 1981). Family members prefer to assume the care of the elderly in the home. A daughter rather than a son is expected to provide major care of ill and aging relatives.

CHILD REARING

First-generation immigrant women have had more children than other Americans. However, second-generation Italian women have curtailed their number of children to a level below that of Americans of native parentage. Third-generation Italian Americans report fewer children still. This trend to smaller family size evolves from the traditional primary concern for the family well-being and continues despite the fact that most Italians are Catholic (Squire & Quadagno, 1988). Italian mothers now favor smaller families. Italian Americans use birth control methods other than rhythm, at a greater rate than other Catholics (Squier & Quadagno, 1988).

Unlike many Caucasian Protestants who generally raise their children to be independent and emphasize self-sufficiency, Italian Americans raise their children to be mutually supportive and faithful to the family. Separation from the family is undesirable and not easily accepted by other members (Rotunno & McGoldrick, 1982). Although individuals of recent generations and those of higher socioeconomic levels value education, the early Italian immigrants often kept their children away from schools to prevent exposure to the influence of outsiders (Squier & Quadagno, 1988).

Italian-American families use discipline frequently. The discipline is usually physical and immediate. Love and affection between parents and children are often employed to help manage and control the children's behavior. Thus, the use of both love and punishment as forms of social control reinforces solidarity and discourages autonomy and independence. A disobedient child is of concern to the entire kin network (Johnson, 1978; Squier & Quadagno, 1988).

Traditional Italian families display a role differentiation between boys and girls. Sons are given much more freedom, permitted some acting-out behavior, and encouraged to develop proficiency in sexual matters essential to the masculine image. Italian males are taught to control their emotions, especially in the presence of outsiders, not necessarily to avoid embarrassment but to prevent harmful exposure to outsiders. On the other hand, girls are allowed to express their emotions freely and are usually more restricted than boys. Girls are given more supervision and guidance and taught to subordinate personal achievements and desires to the service of their parents. They are also taught to keep out of ''men's business'' (Rotunno & McGoldrick, 1982).

SOCIALIZATION PATTERNS

Family solidarity is a basic code for many Italian Americans (Bowen, 1991; Squier & Quadagno, 1988). Italian Americans generally stress the importance of having a good reputation and preserving the family's honor. Men are responsible for maintaining the family's honor, which may involve preventing sexual "misconduct" of the women. Most Italians focus on a positive self-presentation in terms of physical appearance, attire, personality, etiquette, and hospitality. Creating a good impression, *bella figura* (good illustration), is important (Mazur, 1987). Some Italian Americans manifest an external locus of control; that is, their behavior is most often motivated by external factors (Bowen, 1991).

RELIGIOUS BELIEFS AND PRACTICES

Most Italians are Roman Catholic. Although Italians are loyal to the Catholic church, they do not demonstrate leadership in proportion to their numbers. The number of Italian priests remains small (Nelli, 1985).

CULTURALLY BASED HEALTH BELIEFS AND PRACTICES

Generally Italian Americans perceive health in a functional framework; health is a state of optimum ability to perform one's roles and tasks. Some perceive health as a state of well-being that is influenced by age. Aches and pains are expected after age 40. Thus, older people tend to evaluate their health in relation to their capacity to perform normal activities of daily living and maintain physical mobility, whereas some younger people appraise their health by the presence or absence of symptoms (Ragucci, 1981).

Italians Americans usually believe that health maintenance is highly related to proper diet. A good meal is often considered therapy for both emotional and physical problems. Many believe that hard bread and fruit are essential to prevent tooth decay, and the foods most closely related to health preservation are pasta, wine (even for children), salads, fruit, cheese, and home-grown vegetables (Bowen, 1991).

In order to understand the variability in Italian-American beliefs and practices, Ragucci (1981) compared older members (immigrant and second generation) to younger adults. He found that in general the older individuals retained traditional health beliefs, whereas the younger individuals ascribed to the more popular mainstream biomedical beliefs. Italian-American beliefs about illness tend to focus on five factors (although believers in traditional and popular categories differ in the degree of acceptance):

1. *Winds, air currents, and drafts.* Older Italian Americans may show more concern for drafts and air currents than younger individuals. Older persons more often refrain

from using air-conditioners and fans. They may also believe that surgery for cancer will hasten the person's death because of the entrance of air into the body through the incision. Drafts are believed to cause "cold" conditions, referred to as *raffreddore*. Thus, some Italian Americans may refer to upper respiratory infections, muscle pains, or symptoms of gastrointestinal upset as a "cold." For example, nausea and vomiting may be described as a cold in the stomach, and arthritis pain or bursitis in a shoulder would be cold in the shoulder.

2. *Cold and contamination.* Food is never accepted from neighbors or acquaintances whose homes are considered unclean. Nor are visits made to homes of poor house-keepers. Older Italian Americans intensely fear communicable diseases, perhaps influenced by their experience with many diseases before immunization and antibiotics (Ragucci, 1981).

3. *Genes and hereditary factors.* Congenital and hereditary conditions are associated with "blood," which older Italian Americans relate to physical and moral disorders (including behavior problems). Blood conditions may be categorized as "weak," "strong," "good," "bad," "hot," "cold."

4. *Human and supernatural forces.* In addition to iatrogenic causes, humans may cause disease through *malocchio* (evil eye) or by *castiga* (curse). Short-term illnesses like headache or joint pains may be of natural origin or caused by *malocchio*, whereas long-term or possibly fatal illnesses may be attributed to the more powerful *castiga*. *Castiga* are sent by God or an evil person. A *castiga* from God is usually a punishment for some immoral behavior. Diseases such as diabetes, tuberculosis, and cancer were at one time interpreted as punishments (Ragucci, 1981). Because of the strong-weak dichotomy associated with the belief in the *malocchio*, women (especially when pregnant) and children are more susceptible to harm than adult males (Pasquale, 1984). Envy is the emotion that activates the evil eye. Thus, a believer in this phenomenon may perceive a certain illness as resulting from the gaze (eyes) of an envious person. As a precaution against the evil eye, some Italians wear a fist with index and small fingers extended (*mano cornuta*) or a goat's horn (*corno*), made of gold, coral, or plastic (Moss, 1976). An *ittaturi* is a person considered to have the power of *malocchio*, and so this person is avoided by pregnant women and women with small children in the community (Pasquale, 1984).

5. *Psychosomatic factors.* Italian Americans often somatize, yet are aware of the relationships of emotional and physical health. Thus, many acknowledge the ill effects of suppressing emotions with possible consequences of heart disease, hypertension, ulcers, and depression. The Italian expression *sfogare o schiattare* (give vent to emotions or burst) is frequently used to convey an awareness of the therapeutic effect of expressing feelings and not holding things in (Ragucci, 1981).

When ill, many Italians tend to present symptoms in an expressive, dramatic, and detailed manner (Ragucci, 1981; Koopman, Eisenthal & Stoeckle, 1984). Particular attention may focus on the abnormal functioning of the gastrointestinal tract and the liver. Treatment for illness varies from home remedies to the lay referral system to seeking out professional health care. However, professional care is usually sought earlier for a child than for an adult (Ragucci, 1981). Kraut

(1990) noted that many new immigrants appeared to distrust physicians, and when they did visit a health professional, they expected fast results.

When ethnic groups were compared with respect to pain intensity, interference with work and social activities, degree of emotional and psychological stress, and pain expressiveness, Italian Americans were found to indicate the second highest mean scores in these categories (Hispanics were highest). Thus, Italian Americans often experience and report a high intensity of pain due to an intense pain perception, promoting a high degree of emotional stress and interference with work and social activities (Bates & Edwards, 1992).

Folk beliefs and practices include the following:

- Reaching during pregnancy can cause fetal injury and/or deformities.
- Unsatisfied food cravings (*voglie*) can cause fetal anomalies.
- If a pregnant woman smells food that she is not offered, the fetus will move inside and cause a miscarriage. Therefore, neighborhood Italian women always offer food they are cooking to a pregnant woman (Ragucci, 1981).
- Garlic cloves on a string around the neck of an infant or child will prevent colds and "evil stares" from other people that could cause headaches and/or pain in the back and neck. A piece of red ribbon or cloth on an infant could serve the same purpose.
- Placing a scissors under the mattress of a newborn will keep away evil spirits.
- If a woman goes into labor 2 weeks early, she will have a girl and 2 weeks late a boy.
- Never wash hair or bathe during a menstural period.
- To relieve nausea and other stomach ailments, take hot tea, hot ginger ale, castor oil, potato, or baking soda (Spector, 1991).

CULTURAL DIETARY PATTERNS

Being a good cook is a highly rated asset for an Italian wife. Family traditions are strong with respect to holidays, weddings, and funerals, and these occasions are celebrated with food as the central feature. At festive events, Italians may eat for hours, having one special course after another. Wines often accompany the meals. However, Italians have a low rate of alcoholism because drinking is usually done with a meal at the family table (Rotunno & McGoldrick, 1982).

Italian culture is well known for its cuisine. Wine, tomato puree, olive oil, and garlic are favorite seasonings. Some Italian specialties are *polenta* (popular in northern Italy), made with cornmeal and served with a sauce of sausage, other meats, and cheese; *cappelletti*, a dish of small ravioli shaped like hats and filled with different meats and served with chicken broth or sauce; and *gnocchi*, made with mashed potato and served with sauce. Meat sauces are popular and often require six to eight hours of cooking (Bowen, 1991).

Diets considered healthy by Italian Americans contain salads, vegetables, and fresh fruits. Milk is generally not included in the diet. A lactose intolerance has been noted in some Italians (Bozzani, Penagini & Velio, 1986). Italian Americans may have difficulty adhering to therapeutic diets. Because of the importance of food in Italian culture, family, friends, and neighbors often bring gifts of food for a sick person.

MORBIDITY AND MORTALITY

Diseases of genetic origin commonly seen among Italian Americans are favism and the thalassemia syndromes. Favism is a severe hemolytic anemia caused by eating fava beans and the deficiency of an X-linked enzyme. Thalassemia syndromes include Cooley's anemia and alpha thalassemia (Ragucci, 1981).

Some Italian Americans have a problem with lactose intolerance. This has been related to complaints of irritable bowel syndrome in some clients (Bozzani, Penagini & Velio, 1986).

Translations of Some Common Italian Terms

English	Italian
Yes	*Sì*
No	*No*
Nurse	*Infermiera*
Thank you	*Grazie*
Priest	*Sacerdote*
Husband	*Marito*
Wife	*Moglie*
Mother	*Madre*
Father	*Padre*
Son	*Figlio*
Daughter	*Figlia*
Social worker	*Assistente sociale*
Psychologist	*Psicologo*
Pain	*Dolore*
Hot	*Caldo*
Cold	*Freddo*
Numb	*Insensibilità*
Hungry	*Fame*
Thirsty	*Sete*
Short of breath	*Mancanza di fiato*
Allergic	*Allergico*
Food	*Cibo*
Medicine	*Medicine*

Urinal	*Orinale*
Bedpan	*Padella*
Oxygen	*Ossigeno*
Bath	*Fare il bagno*
Blanket	*Coperta*
Water	*Acqua*
Coffee	*Caffè*
Tissues	*Fazzoletto di carta*
Dentures	*Dentiera*
Money	*Denaro*
Leave me alone.	*Milasci solo.*
No visitors	*Nessuna visita*
Get out of bed	*Scendere dal letto*
Back to bed	*Ritornare a letto*
Sit down	*Si sieda in poltrona*
Walk	*Camminare*
Go home	*Andare a casa*
TV	*TV*
Radio	*Radio*
On	*Acceso*
Off	*Spento*
Change	*Cambiare canale-stazione*

Source: Beamatic Communicator. Courtesy of Omnimed Inc., Pine Avenue, P.O. Box 446, Maple Shade, NJ 08052-0446.

REFERENCES

Arenson, S. J. (1979). Rankings of intimacy of social behaviors by Italians and Americans. *Psychological Reports, 44,* 1149–50.

Bates, M. S., & Edwards, W. T. (1992). Ethnic variations in the chronic pain experience. *Ethnicity and Disease, 2*(1), 63–83.

Bowen, M. (1991). Italian Americans. In J. N. Giger & R. E. Davidhizar (Eds.), *Transcultural nursing: Assessment and intervention* (pp. 293–333). St. Louis: Mosby Year Book.

Bozzani, A., Penagini, R., & Velio, P. (1986). Lactose malabsorption and intolerance in Italians. *Digestive Diseases and Sciences, 31*(12), 1313–16.

Bureau of the Census. (1992). *Statistical abstract of the United States.* Washington, DC: Government Printing Office.

Bureau of the Census. (1981). *Statistical reports*. Washington, DC: Government Printing Office.

Cacciola, E. J. (1982). Ethnic and cultural variations in the care of the aged: Some aspects of working with the Italian elderly. *Journal of Geriatric Psychiatry, 15*(2), 197–208.

Daniels, R. (1990). *Coming to America: A history of immigration and ethnicity in American life*. New York: HarperCollins.

Giger, J. N., & Davidhizar, R. E. (1991). *Transcultural nursing: Assessment and intervention*. St. Louis: Mosby Year Book.

Ianni, P. A., & Ruess-Ianni, E. (1972). *A family business: Kinship and social control in organized crime*. New York: Russell Sage.

Johnson, C. L. (1978). Family support systems of elderly Italian Americans. *Journal of Minority Aging, 3–4*, 34–40.

Koopman E., Eisenthal, S., & Stoeckle, J. (1984). Ethnicity in the reported pain, emotional distress and requests of medical outpatients. *Social Science and Medicine, 189*(8), 487–90.

Kraut, A. M. (1990, April 4). Healers and stranger: Immigrant attitudes toward the physician in America, a relationship in historical perspective. *JAMA, 263*(13).

Moss, L. W., & Cappannari, S. C. (1976). Mal occhio, Ayin ha ra, Oculus fascinus, Judenblick: The eye hovers above. In C. Maloney (Ed.), *The evil eye* (pp. 1–16). New York: Columbia University Press.

Nelli, H. S. (1985). Italian Americans in contemporary America. In L. F. Tomasi (Ed.), *Italian Americans: New perspectives in Italian immigration and ethnicity* (pp. 78–87). New York: Center for Migration Studies.

Newman Giger, J., & Davidhizar, R. (1990). Transcultural nursing assessment: A method of advancing nursing practice. *International Nursing Review, 37*(1), 199–202.

Pasquale, E. A. (1984, May–June). The evil eye phenomenon: Its implications for community health nursing. *Home Healthcare Nurse*, pp. 32–35.

Ragucci, A. (1981). Italian Americans. In A. Harwood (Ed.), *Ethnicity and medical care*. Cambridge: Harvard University Press.

Rotunno, M., & McGoldrick, M. (1982). Italian families. In M. McGoldrick, J. K. Pearce & J. Giordano (Eds.), *Ethnicity and family therapy* (pp. 340–63). New York: Guilford Press.

Spector, R. (1991). *Cultural diversity in health and illness* (3d ed.). East Norwalk, CT: Appleton & Lange.

Squier, D. A., & Quadagno, J. S. (1988). The Italian American family. In C. H. Mindel, R. W. Haberstein & R. Wright, Jr. (Eds.), *Ethnic families in America: Patterns and variations* (3d ed.) (pp. 109–37). New York: Elsevier.

Watson, O. M. (1970). *Proxemic behavior: A cross-cultural study*. The Hague, Paris: Mouton.

11

Japanese Americans

Japan, meaning "land of the rising sun," is an island nation located in the north Pacific Ocean off the northeast coast of mainland Asia. The Japanese islands face the former Soviet Union, Korea, and China to the west. The climate of Japan varies depending on latitude. Southwestern Japan experiences long, hot summers and short, cool winters. Northern Japan has short, warm summers and long, cold winters. Typhoons are common during autumn (Pyle, Robinson, & Rubin, 1991).

POPULATION IN THE UNITED STATES

Japanese comprise the third largest Asian group (after Chinese and Filipinos) in the United States, numbering about 850,000 individuals, or approximately 0.3% of the American population. Most Japanese Americans reside on the West Coast (72%), with smaller populations in the South (11%), Northeast (9%), and Midwest (8%). The states with the largest Japanese ancestry population are Hawaii and California (Bureau of the Census, 1992).

IMMIGRATION

Most early Japanese immigrants came to the United States between 1900 and 1924. Their immigration slowed considerably in the 1930s and after 1960 (Daniels, 1990).

After Japan attacked Pearl Harbor during World War II, about 110,000 Japanese (including many who were American citizens), who were residents of the

Pacific states plus 2,000 from Hawaii, were in internment camps. From 1942 to 1945 these camps, enclosed by barbed wire and staffed with armed guards, were located in isolated sites of the West. The internment camps controlled the lives of their Japanese residents (Kitano, 1988; Okamoto, 1978; Sodetani-Shibata, 1981).

COMMUNICATION

Under stress, a Japanese-American client who is fluently bilingual may communicate only in Japanese and require an interpreter similar to some other bilingual individuals. Some Japanese Americans tend to be uncomfortable with sustained direct eye contact (Grippin, 1979).

SOCIOECONOMIC STATUS

The most common Japanese-American employment categories are technical, sales, and administrative support (32%), followed by managerial and professional specialty occupations (29%). Japanese Americans are one of the most economically successful minority groups (Kitano, 1988; Minority Rights Group, 1989). Individuals of higher socioeconomic status generally demonstrate more concern for prevention of illness and maintenance of health than lower-status persons (Chrisman & Kleinman, 1980; Harwood, 1981).

CHIEF COMPLAINT

Many Japanese Americans describe symptoms with less emotion than the average American (Lock, 1983). Some Japanese Americans are extremely sensitive to even minor somatic symptoms. Psychosomatic and nonspecific complaints are frequently presented by individuals seeking health care. However, the health professional should not assume that a symptom is psychosomatic and unrelated to pathology (Lock, 1983). Although some Japanese-American menopausal women show a relatively low incidence of "hot flashes," they tend to present various nonspecific somatic complaints, such as abdominal pains and headache (Lock, 1986).

FAMILY

Japanese Americans are the only ethnic group that has named their generational levels. The first generation (first immigrants to settle in America) is called *Issei*, the second (their offspring) is *Nisei*, and the third generation is known as *Sansei*. The fourth and fifth generations are called the *Yansei* and *Goset*, respectively (Kitano, 1988; Okamoto, 1978).

The traditional Japanese-American family (*Issei*) has the following characteristics:

- Patriarchal, hierarchical structure.
- Emphasis on obedience to elders, filial piety, and rank.
- Interdependence of family members.
- Women subordinate to men.
- Purpose of marriage is to continue the family, and marriage for love is considered immoral because it places personal feelings before the family. Traditional marriages are often parent arranged (Kitano, 1988; Okamoto, 1978).

Most *Nisei* are 50 years of age or older. They are influenced by traditional Japanese family values as well as those of mainstream America. Their families have these characteristics:

- Marriage partners tend to be freely chosen on the basis of romantic love.
- The bond between husband and wife (conjugal bond) takes priority over the bond between parent and child (filial bond).
- The marital relationship is more egalitarian, with greater flexibility of sex roles.
- The emphasis is on upward socioeconomic mobility (Yanagisako, 1985).

The modern *Sansei*, typically born in the United States, comprise the majority of the young adult Japanese-American population. *Sansei* retain some traditional Japanese family values but are more likely to follow American mainstream family practices. The following exemplify some Sansei family values and practices:

- Some *Sansei* select non–Japanese Americans as spouses.
- Attitudes about marriage are closely related to those of most Americans.
- Love is viewed as the most important aspect of marriage.
- The conjugal bond takes precedence over filial bonds and kinship relationships.
- Although some male dominance persists within the family, many *Sansei* couples have adopted an egalitarian model of family relationships.
- Separation and divorce are becoming more common.
- Some families maintain strong identification with the extended family network; hierarchies may persist (Sodetani-Shibata, 1981).
- The mother-in-law and other elders are usually highly influential in making family decisions concerning the client's health care. If the client is a male elder, his son will most likely assume the role of decision maker. If the client is a female elder, her son or husband will probably take responsibility for decisions about her health care (Berlin & Fowkes, 1983).

Some *Nisei* and *Sansei* have demonstrated a high degree of assimilation into American culture as indicated by use of the English language, out-of-group marriages (60–65%), residing outside concentrated Japanese areas, high educational levels, and a wide range of professional occupations (Kitano, 1988; Lock, 1983). The *Sansei, Yansei,* and *Goset* are probably most amenable to American mainstream medical practices.

ELDERLY

Japanese families usually prefer to have their elderly cared for by a family member (*miuchi*) rather than by an unrelated person (*tanin*) (Inoue, 1983). Dependent Japanese-American elders expect to be cared for and therefore readily cooperate with caretakers in the home as well as in the hospital (Hartog & Hartog, 1983).

Findings in a study of nursing homes noted that elderly Japanese Americans (many of whom were born in Japan) placed high emphasis on ethnic factors of the environment and ethnic homogeneity of the staff. Thus, they tended to prefer Japanese nurses and preferred to receive Japanese meals (Chee & Kane, 1983).

CHILD REARING

The traditional Japanese-American mother usually employs a great deal of nonverbal communication and maintains close physical proximity with her baby. She may rock, soothe, and sleep with her infant, thereby fostering dependency rather than independence. Traditional Japanese mothers usually prefer a quiet and contented baby.

Nisei and *Sansei* mothers demonstrate childbearing behaviors that are somewhere between traditional Japanese and mainstream American practices. *Nisei, Sansei,* and later-generation mothers typically encourage separateness and independence by allowing the infant to sleep in a crib. They often emphasize verbal communication by talking to the baby and encouraging infant expression. *Nisei* and *Sansei* usually desire a more vocal and active baby (Sodetani-Shibata, 1981).

Japanese-American children are taught respect for elders, role conformity, orderliness, tidiness, and good manners. They are expected to be polite, obedient, and concerned about what others think. Children are encouraged to develop a strong sense of commitment and loyalty to their kinship group (Kitano, 1988; Sodetani-Shibata, 1981). Verbal approval or disapproval through the use of guilt or shame is used to maintain discipline. Occasionally, light hitting may be used for punishment (Sodetani-Shibata, 1981).

SOCIALIZATION PATTERNS

Some Japanese Americans may use nonverbal behavior, such as a bowed head, repeated nodding in agreement, and avoidance of sustained eye contact during communication with health professionals. This behavior could be viewed as shyness but may in fact be a method of demonstrating respect for authority.

Some may constantly display an agreeable manner, indicative of a need to maintain harmony in social situations.

A method of coping with stressful situations may be to maintain social harmony and suppress conflict. Health professionals should be aware that some Japanese-American clients might deal with conflict by retreatism (escaping the situation) or ritualism (outwardly conforming by suppressing internal conflict) (Lock, 1983). Because some Japanese Americans have sanctions against verbalizing negative feelings about family members, family counseling and therapy may be problematic (Lock, 1983). Japanese Americans display an underutilization of mental health services. Self and family resources are used most commonly (Uomoto & Gorsuch, 1984).

The term *enryo* encompasses the norms of restraint, reserve, and lack of assertion in social interactions (Kitano, 1988; Sodetani-Shibata, 1981; Yip, Lim & Fung, 1978). A dominant aspect of the Japanese-American personality is the tendency to suppress negative feelings toward others, including family, intimates, and those in authority (Lock, 1983).

The term *amae* means the need to be loved and accepted. *Amae* begins with the infant at the mother's breast and may extend to a continued dependency of some adult children on their parents (Doi, 1973; Shon & Ja, 1982; Sodetani-Shibata, 1981). Because of a tendency to depend on the family, some Japanese Americans will not make an important decision about health care until another family member is consulted first. Hospital consent forms that require the client's signature such as permission for surgery or major treatments should be presented to the client when a family member (particularly the leader) is present. This tendency toward dependency could delay the Japanese-American client's active participation in his or her own health care (Hartog & Hartog, 1983).

Because many Japanese Americans are stoic and display a high pain tolerance level, the health professional should check for noverbal signs of discomfort. Physiological indicators of discomfort could include elevated blood pressure, increased pulse and heart rates, and diaphoresis. The health professional should determine the need for prn pain and sleep medications even when the client has not requested them. Because of this stoic behavior pattern it is necessary to monitor the Japanese-American woman's cervical dilation and rate of contractions carefully on a labor and delivery unit, since she may not indicate progress by expressions of discomfort (Okamoto, 1978).

Because some Japanese Americans tend to refrain from verbally expressing discomfort, the health professional should encourage the client to verbalize more frequently and become less dependent on nonverbal behaviors in the hospital setting. Not speaking up could delay proper health care and thus cause a condition to worsen. For example, not asking for medication until the pain becomes unbearable could diminish the effect of the medication when it is finally administered.

The Japanese-American infant or child client may behave in a quiet manner and seldom cry. Staff should give as much unsolicited attention to this child as time permits. If possible, arrange to have a cot placed in the child's room so that the Japanese-American mother may room in with her sick infant if she desires.

RELIGIOUS BELIEFS AND PRACTICES

The predominant religions in Japan are Shinto and Buddhism, less than 1% of Japan's population practice Christianity (Ensminger, Ensminger, Kolande & Robson, 1983; Pyle et al., 1991). Confucianism, a Chinese philosophy, has greatly influenced Japanese thinking, although it was never strongly organized in Japan (Katagawa, 1988; Miller, 1988; Pyle et al., 1991).

Shinto, the native religion of Japan, is a complex of beliefs, customs, and practices distinguished from the religions of India and China (Buddhism and Confucianism, respectively) (Eliade & Couliano, 1991). Shintoists worship gods and goddesses (*kami*) who are forces of nature residing in trees, rivers, rocks, mountains, the wind, some animals, and particularly the sun and moon (Eliade & Couliano, 1991; Miller, 1988; Seward, 1972). Japanese ancestor worship is basically a Shinto institution, often altered by Confucian and Buddhist rituals. Shinto religion places high value on cleanliness, and therefore many Japanese clients are particular about a clean environment. They believe that cleanliness helps to prevent the spread of communicable diseases.

Buddhism, which developed from the teachings of Guatama Buddha of India, was brought to Japan from China during the sixth century. Buddhism amalgamated with the existing Shinto religion, and its followers practiced Shinto-Buddhism (Katagawa, 1988; Seward, 1972). Buddhism teaches the individual to think more intensely about the meaning of human existence in order to experience intuitive understanding. Buddhism encourages passivity, stoicism, and behavioral reserve (Eliade & Couliano, 1991; Miller, 1988; Seward, 1972). Some Japanese-American Buddhists practice restraint in expressing negative feelings and tend not to complain about uncomfortable situations, such as an unanswered call bell, unappetizing meals, delayed bath, or late medication. Buddhists believe that when a person dies, the individual goes to "the pure land" and is welcomed by Buddha. The deceased then becomes an ancestor with whom the living may maintain contact (Eliade & Couliano, 1991). Consequently, Buddhists tend to have less difficulty than some other individuals in accepting the loss of a loved one due to this expectation of continued contact (Grippin, 1979).

Zen is a form of Buddhism. The term means silent meditation. Zen Buddhism was brought from China and established in Japan by two monks, Eisai and Dogen, during the thirteenth century. Zen emphasizes meditation and enlightenment through intuitive thought, self-discipline, and direct and unhesitating style of life. Because of Zen's focus on direct, unhesitating behavior, this form of Buddhism became popular among the Japanese military (Dumoulin, 1988; Seward, 1972).

CULTURALLY BASED HEALTH BELIEFS AND PRACTICES

Many Japanese Americans believe in the holistic concept of health: all parts of the body are interrelated; the mind and the body are inseparable; and social, psychological, and physiological factors contribute to health and illness. Consequently, many believe that therapy should be directed to the entire body rather than only to the area of complaint and that therapy should also address the social and environmental implications of the condition (Lock, 1980, 1983).

Since many Japanese Americans are future oriented, they tend to practice prevention, such as inoculations, prenatal care, and proper diet. Consequently they are amenable to health education related to health promotion and disease prevention (Hartog & Hartog, 1983).

Some Japanese Americans believe that illness is related to yin or yang states and that a dietary balance between yin and yang is required to maintain health, as well as to treat disease conditions (Chow, 1976; Lock, 1980). The yin state is associated with symptoms of "internal cold" and reduced body function. In contrast, symptoms of the yang state are generalized hyperactivity with external manifestations such as a "warm" sensation and/or an elevated temperature (Lock, 1980). Herbal medicines, despite their bitter taste, are considered harmless, without side effects, and similar to food. Some Japanese-American families ingest herbal liquid mixtures two to four times a day as preventatives (Lock, 1980).

All herbal medications are classified by traditional practitioners according to the yin-yang theory. Yin-type medications have a cooling effect, while yang-type medications warm the body (Lock, 1980). Based on the yin-yang theory, many foods are classified as "hot" or "cold" (unrelated to temperature). Examples of yin (cold) foods are most fresh fruits and vegetables, soybeans, and seaweed. Examples of yang (hot) foods are chicken, beef, red beans, and ginseng. Yin foods are usually bland; yang foods are often spicy. Rice and tea are neutral foods (Andrews, 1989; Burtis, Davis & Martin, 1989; Lock, 1980). Disease conditions are also classified as yin or yang and treated accordingly. For example, a yang (hot) condition, such as a fever or sore throat, could be treated with a yin food or herb. After childbirth, considered a yin (cold) condition, the mother may be given hot (yang) foods for at least a month postpartum (Andrews, 1989; Lock, 1978).

Ginseng or ginseng root (often called the root of life) is a popular herb used by Japanese Americans. Classed as a yang substance, it is often ingested as a rejuvenator by pregnant women, athletes, older persons, or anyone in a "weakened" condition (Andrews, 1989). Adverse reactions associated with the long-term use of ginseng include nervousness, insomnia, edema, or irregularities in blood glucose levels (Ginseng, 1980).

CULTURAL DIETARY PATTERNS

Rice is the staple food of the Japanese diet and is served with almost every meal. Fish and soybean products are major sources of dietary protein. Soybean curd (tofu) is used extensively. Japanese Americans usually eat less meat and more vegetables than other Americans. Fresh vegetables are slightly cooked (often stir fried) to preserve crispness and nutrients. Edible seaweed is popular in Japanese cuisine.

Japanese Americans prefer their food chopped in small pieces that are easier to manage with chopsticks. Favorite deserts are fruits, especially melons, berries, and tangerines (Burtis, Davis & Martin, 1989; Tien-Hyatt, 1987). Tea is the favorite beverage. Sake, a rice wine, is a popular alcoholic drink (Ensminger et al., 1983).

Strict Buddhists are vegetarians. They avoid eating the flesh of any animal (except fish), as well as milk and eggs. They also abstain from alcoholic beverages. The limitations of a vegetarian diet are significant during periods when the body has high protein requirements, such as infancy, growth, stress, surgery, and illness. Inadequate dietary protein could delay healing, compromise the immune system, and slow the growth rate for a child (Burtis, Davis & Martin, 1988). Benefits of a vegetarian diet include better weight control, less constipation, lower blood pressure, and decreased incidence of conditions such as gallstones, colon cancer, and breast cancer (Burtis, Davis & Martin, 1988).

Careful planning is required to maintain proper daily levels of amino acids necessary to build protein. Various combinations of protein-containing foods should be used to complement one another, such as grains and legumes (rice and beans, corn soy bread), legumes and nuts (roasted soybean snacks with bean soup), and grains and nuts (rice and cashews). Since Vitamin B12 is available only in animal products, B12 supplements should be added to the strict vegetarian's diet. In addition, iron and calcium supplements are recommended for the strict vegetarian woman during pregnancy (Burtis, Davis & Martin, 1988).

MORBIDITY AND MORTALITY

Japanese Americans of both sexes have one of the longest life expectancies of any other large population subgroup in the United States (Curb, Reed, Miller & Yano, 1990). Between 1972 and 1982, Japan reached and surpassed Sweden's record as the country with the longest life expectancy (Yanagishita & Guralnik, 1988).

Lactose enzyme deficiency is found in about 90% of Japanese-American adults. Individuals with this condition are unable to digest the lactose in milk and other dairy products. Symptoms of lactose intolerance include gastrointestinal upset, cramping, and diarrhea. If lactose intolerance is a problem, inform the client and family about lactose-free products found in the dairy section of food stores and Lactaid (lactase enzyme) drops or caplets available in drug stores. Cheese aged over 60 days may be eaten because lactose is converted to lactic acid during the aging process (Burtis, Davis & Martin, 1988).

Because feelings are not readily expressed, Japanese Americans often convert their emotions into somatic conditions, which are brought to the attention of the health provider. They are vulnerable to stress-related illnesses (Grippin, 1979; Lock, 1983).

Japanese-American women were found to have a lower rate of breast cancer than Caucasian women but a 3.5 times higher rate of breast cancer than their peers in Japan. These findings indicate that environmental factors play a larger role than genetic factors in determining breast cancer risk (Nomura, Lee, Kolonel & Hirohata, 1984; Shimizu, Ross, Bernstein & Yatani, 1991).

Mortality rates of coronary heart disease are much lower in Japanese Americans than in Caucasians, but hemorrhagic stroke rates are higher in Japanese Americans than in Caucasians. Plasma fibrinogen levels and coagulation factors were found to be significantly higher in Caucasians than in Japanese-Americans. This may partly explain the difference in mortality from cardiovascular disease between these two populations. These differences may be related to diet and genetics (Iso, Folson, Wu & Finch, 1989).

There is a significant positive relationship between coffee consumption and serum cholesterol. This relationship is not present with other sources of caffeine such as tea and cola. Thus, tea drinkers tend to have lower serum cholesterol levels than coffee drinkers. Tea is usually the preferred beverage among Japanese Americans (Curb, Reed, Kautz & Yano, 1986).

Cancer of the digestive organs appears to be more prevalent in Japanese Americans than in Caucasians. However, in general Japanese Americans have a lower incidence of other cancers.

Japanese Americans tend to have a slightly higher incidence of diabetes and pneumonia than Caucasians. Their most common health problems are peptic ulcer, hypertension, arthritis, diabetes, and gout.

Older age groups (ages 75–81) have a higher incidence of heart disease and stroke (Curb, Reed, Miller & Yano, 1990; Gerber, 1983; Park, Yokoyama, & Tokuyama 1991; Peterson, Rose & McGee, 1985). Among Japanese Americans, arteriosclerotic disease ranks highest as a cause of death, followed by COPD, infection, and diabetes (Park, Yokoyama & Tokuyama, 1991).

Coronary occlusion is the major cause of sudden death among Japanese Americans. Although the incidence of stroke is high, it is not the major cause of sudden death (Yano, McCarthy, Reed & Kagan, 1987).

BELIEFS ABOUT DEATH AND DYING

Some Japanese-American clients and families may avoid discussions related to impending death because they believe that nonverbal methods are the most effective means of communicating feelings (Lock, 1983). Some may express grief by developing somatic ailments (Lawson, 1990). According to Buddhist philosophy, an individual's mind should be calm, hopeful, and clear at the time of death in order to reincarnate into a better person. Thus, a dying client or the client's family might refuse medication that could alter consciousness (Tien-Hyatt, 1987).

PHYSICAL ASSESSMENT

Generally, Japanese Americans tend to be shorter than the average American (Overfield, 1985). They tend to have a lower bone mineral content than Caucasians of the same sex and age, which may account for their smaller body size (Yano, Wasnich, Vogel & Heilbrun, 1984). Therefore American mainstream growth and development standards for use in physically assessing Japanese-American children are inappropriate because they tend to be normally smaller in body structure and less active than Caucasian children (Caudill & Frost, 1972).

The epicanthic fold of the eyelids, a vertical fold found at the inner corners of the eyes, causes the eyes to appear far apart. This is a normal finding among Japanese Americans (Miller & Keane, 1987).

Some individuals tend to have large teeth that give a definite shape to the jaw. The eruption of teeth may normally occur earlier in Japanese-American infants than in Caucasian infants (Chang, 1981).

REFERENCES

Andrews, M. M. (1989). Culture and nutrition. In J. S. Boyle & M. M. Andrews (Eds.), *Transcultural concepts in nursing care* (pp. 333–55). Glenview, IL: Scott, Foresman/Little, Brown.

Berlin, E. A., & Fowkes, W. C., Jr. (1983). A teaching framework for cross-cultural health care. *Western Journal of Medicine, 139*(6), 934–38.

Bureau of the Census. (1990). *U.S. Department of Commerce News*. Washington, DC: Government Printing Office.

Burtis, G., Davis, J., & Martin, S. (1989). *Applied nutrition and diet therapy*. Philadelphia: W. B. Saunders Company.

Caudill, W., & Frost, N. (1972). A comparison of maternal care and infant behavior in Japanese-American, American, and Japanese families. In U. Bronfenbrenner & M. Mahoney (Eds.), *Influences on health development*. Fort Worth, TX: Dryden Press.

Chang, B. (1981). Asian American patient care. In G. Henderson & M. Primeaux (Eds.), *Transcultural health care* (pp. 255–78). Reading, MA: Addison-Wesley.

Chee, P., & Kane, R. (1983). Cultural factors affecting nursing home care for minorities: A study of black American and Japanese-American groups. *Journal of the American Geriatrics Society, 31*(2), 109–12.

Chow, E. (1976). Cultural health traditions: Asian perspectives. In M. F. Branch & P. P. Paxton (Eds.), *Providing safe nursing care for ethnic people of color* (pp. 99–114). New York: Appleton-Century-Crofts.

Chrisman, N. J., & Kleinman, A. (1980). Health beliefs and practices. In S. Thernstrom (Ed.), *Harvard encyclopedia of American ethnic groups* (pp. 452–61). Cambridge: Belknap Press of Harvard University Press.

Curb, J. D., Reed, D. M., Kautz, J. A., & Yano, K. (1986). Coffee, caffeine, and serum cholesterol in Japanese men in Hawaii. *American Journal of Epidemiology, 123*(4), 648–55.

Curb, J. D., Reed, D. M., Miller, F. D., & Yano, K. (1990). Health style in elderly Japanese men with a long life expectancy. *Journal of Gerontology, 45*(5), 5206–11.

Doi, T. (1973). *The anatomy of dependence.* New York: Harper & Row.

Dumoulin, H. (1988). Zen. In M. Eliade (Ed.), *The encyclopedia of religion* (Vol. 15) (pp. 561–68). New York: Macmillan.

Eliade, M., & Couliano, I. P. (1991). *The Eliade guide to world religions.* San Francisco: Harper.

Ensminger, A. H., Ensminger, M. E., Kolande, J. E., & Robson, R. K. (1983). *Foods and nutrition encyclopedia* (Vols. 1 & 2). Clovis, CA: Pegus Press.

Gerber, L. M. (1983). Gains in life expectancies if heart disease and stroke were eliminated among Caucasians, Filipinos and Japanese in Hawaii. *Social Science Medicine, 17*(6), 349–53.

Ginseng. (1980). *Medical Letter Drugs Therapy, 22*(17), 72.

Grippin, J. T. (1979). The Japanese American client. *Issues in Mental Health Nursing, 2*(1), 57–69.

Hartog, J., & Hartog, E. A. (1983). Cultural aspects of health and illness behavior in hospitals. *Western Journal of Medicine, 136*(6), 910–15.

Harwood, A. (1981). Guidelines for culturally appropriate health care. In A. Harwood (Ed.), *Ethnicity and medical care* (pp. 482–508). Cambridge: Harvard University Press.

Inoue, I. (1983). Attendance care at hospitals in Japan. *International Nursing Review, 32*(2), 172–17.

Iso, H., Folsom, A. R., Wu, K. K., & Finch, A. (1989). Hemostatic variables in Japanese and Caucasian men: Plasma fibrinogen, factor VIIc, factor VIIIc, and von Willebrand factor and their relations to cardiovascular disease risk factors. *American Journal of Epidemiology, 130*(5), 925–34.

Katagawa, J. M. (1988). Japanese religion: An overview. In M. Eliade (Ed.), *The encyclopedia of religion* (Vol. 7) (pp. 520–38). New York: Macmillan.

Kitano, H. L. (1988). The Japanese American family. In C. H. Mindel, R. W. Haberstein & R. Wright, Jr., *Ethnic families in America* (3d ed.) (pp. 258–75). New York: Elsevier.

Koschmann, V. J. (1978). *Authority and the individual in Japan: Citizen protest in historical perspective.* Tokyo: University of Tokyo Press.

Lawson, L. V. (1990). Culturally sensitive support for grieving parents. *Maternal and Child Nursing, 15*, 76–79.

Lock, M. M. (1980). An examination of the influence of traditional therapeutic systems on the practice of cosmopolitan medicine in Japan. *American Journal of Chinese Medicine, 8*(3), 221–29.

Lock, M. M. (1983). Cross-cultural medicine: Japanese responses to social change; making the strange familiar. *Western Journal of Medicine, 139*(6), 829–34.

Lock, M. M. (1986). Ambiguities of aging: Japanese experience and perceptions of menopause. *Culture and Medical Psychiatry, 10*(1), 23–46.

Miller, A. L. (1988). Japanese religion: Popular religions. In M. Eliade (Ed.), *The encyclopedia of religion* (Vol. 7) (pp. 538–44). New York: Macmillan.

Miller, B. F., & Keane, C. B. (1987). *Encyclopedia and dictionary of medicine, nursing, and allied health.* Philadelphia: W. B. Saunders.

Minority Rights Group. (1989). *World dictionary of minorities: St. James international references.* Chicago: St. James Press.

Nomura, A. M., Lee, J., Kolonel, L. N., & Hirohata, T. (1984). Breast cancer in two populations with different levels of risk for the disease. *American Journal of Epidemiology, 119*(4), 496–502.

Okamoto, N. I. (1978). The Japanese American. In A. L. Clark (Ed.), *Culture childbearing health professionals.* Philadelphia: F. A. Davis Co.

Overfield, T. (1985). *Biological variations in health and illness: Race, age and sex differences.* Reading, MA: Addison-Wesley.

Park, C. B., Yokoyama, E., & Tokuyama, G. H. (1991). Medical conditions at death among Caucasian and Japanese elderly in Hawaii: Analysis of multiple causes of death, 1976–78. *Journal of Clinical Epidemiology, 44*(6), 519–30.

Peterson, M. R., Rose, C. L., & McGee, R. I. (1985). A cross-cultural study of Japanese elders in Hawaii. *International Journal of Aging and Human Development, 21*(4), 267–79.

Pyle, K. B., Robinson, M., & Rubin, J. (1991). Japan. *The world book encyclopedia.* Chicago: Scott Fetzer Co.

Seward, J. (1972). *The Japanese.* New York: William Morrow.

Shimizu, H., Ross, R. K., Berstein, L., & Yatani, R. (1991). Cancers of the prostate and breast among Japanese and white immigrants in Los Angeles County. *British Journal of Cancer, 63*(6), 963–66.

Shon, S. P., & Ja, D. Y. (1982). Asian families. In M. McGoldrick, J. P. Pearce & J. Giordano, (Eds.), *Ethnicity and family therapy* (pp. 208–28). New York: Guilford Press.

Sodetani-Shibata, A. E. (1981). The Japanese American. In A. L. Clark (Ed.), *Culture childrearing* (pp. 96–138). Philadelphia: F. A. Davis Co.

Stavig, G. R., Igra, A., & Leonard, A. R. (1988). Hypertension and related health issues among Asians and Pacific Islanders in California. *Public Health Reports, 103*(10), 28–37.

Tien-Hyatt, J. L. (1987). Keying in on the unique care needs of Asian clients. *Nursing and Health Care, 8*(5), 268–71.

Uomoto, J. M., & Gorsuch, R. L. (1984). Japanese American responses to psychological disorder: Referral patterns attitudes, and subjective norms. *American Journal of Community Psychology, 12*(5), 537–50.

Yanagisako, S. J. (1985). *Transforming the past.* Stanford, CA: Stanford University Press.

Yanagishita, M., & Guralnik, J. M. (1988). Changing mortality patterns that led life expectancy in Japan to surpass Sweden's; 1972–1982. *Demography, 25*(4), 611–24.

Yano, K., McCarthy, L. J., Reed, D. M., & Kagan, A. (1987). Postmortem findings in sudden death and non–sudden death among Japanese-American men in Hawaii. *American Journal of Medicine, 86*(6), 1036–44.

Yano, K., Wasnich, R. D., Vogel, J. M., & Heilbrun, L. K. (1984). Bone mineral measurements among middle aged and elderly Japanese residents in Hawaii. *American Journal of Epidemiology, 119*(5), 751–64.

Yip, B. C., Lim, H., & Fung, V. H. (1978). *Understanding the Pan Asian client.* San Diego, CA: Union of Pan Asian Communities.

12

Jewish Americans

Jewish Americans are difficult to describe because of their diverse origins. Yet Jews have retained a high degree of religious and cultural identity. They have been a group on the move with thousands of years of history yet with no single country of origin. Jews have migrated to America from many countries, including Spain, Portugal, Germany, Poland, Russia, Rumania, Hungary, Austria, Lithuania, and Asia (Farber, Mindel, & Lazerwitz, 1988; Hertz & Rosen, 1982; Schwartz, 1991).

POPULATION IN THE UNITED STATES

Jewish Americans constitute about 3% of the American population (Schwartz, 1991). Calculated by temple membership, there are approximately 6 million Jewish Americans in the United States (Bureau of the Census, 1992). The majority of Jewish Americans appear to have congregated on the East and West coasts of the United States, with the largest percentages residing in New York, California, Pennsylvania, Illinois, and Florida (Bureau of the Census, 1992).

IMMIGRATION

Historically, there were three major waves of Jewish migrations to America, with some overlapping of these groups. Sephardic Jews, originally from Spain and Portugal, formed the earliest Jewish settlement in New Amsterdam in 1654. German Jews, a larger group, migrated from about 1840 to 1880, after conditions in Bavaria placed many restrictions on the Jewish people. East European Jews, originally from Poland, Russia, Rumania, Hungary, and Lithuania, began arriving in the 1880s, and their descendants now constitute about 90% of American Jews (Farber, Mindel & Lazerwitz, 1988). Immigration was instigated by imperial Russia's pogroms, attacks of violence on the towns and villages of Russia.

In contrast, the earlier Jewish immigrants came from cultures into which they had integrated, and they generally settled in nonsegregated sections in America. On the other hand, the East European Jews came from areas where they were isolated and limited to the Jewish community. In these predominantly Jewish villages, there was little if any integration, so the strong Jewish culture was unaffected by the cultures around them. This Jewish community was called the *shtetl* (Farber, Mindel & Lazerwitz, 1988; Schwartz, 1991).

Jews experienced a somewhat different immigration pattern from that of many other immigrants. Although many other immigrant individuals might have had a padrone or family facilitator, they did not usually rent from or work for their own ethnic group. Whereas many Jewish immigrants obtained jobs in Jewish-owned factories in the garment districts and lived in tenements, where they paid rent to Jewish landlords (Daniels, 1990).

Jews differed from many other immigrants in their intent to stay in America rather than to earn money and return to their homeland. Jews had only about a 5% remigration rate, of which some emigrated again later. Of all the other ethnic groups, only the Irish had a rate below 10%. Many other East European groups had remigration rates up to 87%. Hence Jews settled in America with a sense of permanence (Daniels, 1990).

COMMUNICATION

Today the principal language of Jewish Americans is English, often sprinkled with some Yiddish expressions (Schwartz, 1991). Traditionally, Yiddish, a German dialect written in Hebrew characters, was the common *mamaloshen* (mother tongue) of most East European Jews. Literate women were taught Yiddish, whereas only men were taught Hebrew (Farber, Mindel & Lazerwitz, 1988). Other major groups of Jews were the Sephardim (from Spain and Portugal) who spoke Ladino, a dialect of Spanish written in Hebrew, and the Asian Jews, who usually used the Arabic language (Farber, Mindel & Lazerwitz, 1988). Hebrew is the language of Israel. Although Hebrew is not spoken by most Jews, many can read it. Hebrew is described by Trepp (1980): "We may pray in any language; yet Hebrew holds a special significance. It is the holy tongue of Torah, the tongue of creation. It is the language in which the covenant was made between Israel and God and among the members of Israel's community themselves" (p. 41).

SOCIOECONOMIC STATUS

Many German-Jewish immigrants started out as foot peddlers who traveled throughout America. Some later acquired horses and wagons and then shops, often dry goods stores. From these ventures evolved some of the great department stores in America (Farber, Mindel & Lazerwitz, 1988).

Many East European Jewish immigrants were tradesmen, dairymen, cobblers, tailors, butchers, peddlers, and shopkeepers (Farber, Mindel & Lazerwitz, 1988). Some Jewish immigrants never worked for others but began as small tradesmen; others left the labor market and often became successful entrepreneurs (Daniels, 1990).

Although Jews make up only 3% of the American population, their achievements are visible in many aspects of America—the arts, academia, sciences, medicine, law, and politics (Schwartz, 1991). Many major Hollywood studios were founded or controlled by dynamic Jewish immigrants (Daniels, 1990). The first birth control clinic was opened in Brownsville, a Jewish community in Brooklyn, New York, by Margaret Sanger (Farber, Mindel & Lazerwitz, 1988). Notable politicians include Ed Koch, former mayor of New York City.

CHIEF COMPLAINT

Many Jewish individuals describe their symptoms in detail. Some Jews are articulate and self-expressive. Thus, responses to questions might offer a great deal of information about pain, illness, interfamily relations, anxieties, and so forth. Dramatic expressions of pain with moaning and crying are not uncommon (Schwartz, 1991). Jewish families are more likely to have mild or moderate neurotic symptoms, compared to the more serious symptoms found in some other cultures, and to seek psychotherapy (Strole, Langer, Michael, Opler & Rennie, 1962).

FAMILY

The relationship of Jewish family life to Jewish religion is documented in the Torah (the five books of Moses), the Talmud (Rabbinic code), and the Mishnah (legal and ethical teachings) (Schlesinger, 1974; Schwartz, 1991; Trepp, 1980).

The Traditional Family

Male dominance and filial responsibility have been characteristics of the traditional Jewish family (Schlesinger, 1974). The father has been the head of the family unit, owner of its property, and highly valued for his public status and financial support (Hertz & Rosen, 1982; Schlesinger, 1974). He has had important responsibilities in the spiritual and intellectual spheres. Traditionally, only men were taught to read, write, and speak Hebrew. The father has had a priestly role in the household, responsible for the morality and ethical standards of the family members, a link between the family and the religious community (Farber, Mindel & Lazerwitz, 1988).

Despite her subordination to the father, the mother has maintained a position of honor and authority in the family. Her responsibility has been to care for the home, the children and her husband (Schlesinger, 1974). She has sometimes been viewed as overbearing and/or overprotective (Schwartz, 1991).

The family structure, generally nuclear, has often been three generational and included grandparents. The *shtetl* was perceived as the extended family (Farber, Mindel & Lazerwitz, 1988).

In Eastern Europe, marriages were arranged by the parents of the couple or the marriage broker (*shadken*). The purposes of marriage were companionship and procreation. *Kiddushin*, the Hebrew term for marriage, was interpreted as "the state of holiness." The divorce rate among Jewish couples has been low (Hertz & Rosen 1982; Schlesinger, 1974).

Intermarriage was unpopular and perceived as a betrayal of the family and community. Consequently, emotional cutoffs were not uncommon. In such a cutoff, the family would "sit shiva," a seven-day period of mourning for a member who intermarried (Gordon, 1964).

Within the family, the mother often appeared to be more demonstratively affectionate to her sons, whereas the father was more demonstrative toward his daughters (Farber, Mintz & Lazerwitz, 1988).

Traditional Jewish family life can be summarized as patriarchal, three-generational, symbolic of continuity of life and a measure of timelessness, embodying wholeness of life, embracing birth, education, marriage, sickness, and celebrations embodying religion and its related activities, and serving as a learning environment with emphasis on the pursuit of learning.

The Modern Family

Although Jewish Americans have a relatively high fertility rate, there has been a recent reduction in the number of children in families. Jewish Americans have been quite successful with regard to family planning and birth control.

Marriages are no longer arranged. Intermarriages and the divorce rate have increased (Farber, Mintz & Lazerwitz, 1988).

Rather than generational divisions to determine adherence to traditional customs, Jewish Americans are generally categorized with respect to denominational preferences: Orthodox, Conservative, or Reform.

Orthodox Jews, 11% of the adult Jewish population, attempt to carry out traditional Jewish religious practices and values into modern life with as few changes as possible. Highly Orthodox Jews are easily recognized. The men usually have long earlocks and beards. They wear either skull caps or large black hats, and long black coats. The women usually dress modestly in long-sleeved dresses, with wigs or scarves covering their heads (Schwartz, 1991).

Conservative Jews, 40% of the American Jewish population, generally practice some balance between religious/traditional and modern practices.

Reform Jews, 30% of American Jews, have abandoned many religious and traditional practices.

Finally, about 19% of the American Jewish population view themselves as "just Jewish" and may be marginal to the Jewish community and its religious practices (Farber, Mindel & Lazerwitz, 1988).

CHILD REARING

The birth of a child is considered a blessing. A child represents continuation of the Jewish culture. Thus, education of the child with respect to Jewish customs is extremely important (Schlesinger, 1974).

Jewish-American parents tend to be permissive, overprotective, and deeply concerned about their children's future happiness. Children are viewed as individuals with unique drives that require both outlets and controls. Parents use reasoning, explanation, and rationality. Punishment is a means of diverting behavior into more acceptable channels (Hertz & Rosen, 1982). Channeling of behavior in Jewish-American families means that each year, the child must assume new responsibilities, such as helping with the younger ones, going to *cheder* (religious school), becoming a scholar, earning a living, and so forth.

Through the rituals of daily prayers, Jewish-American children are usually taught to delay gratification, use sublimation rather than inhibition, and rely on authority and benefice rather than reciprocity to justify behavior (Farber, Mindel & Lazerwitz, 1988).

Major Life Stages

Stages of life are usually acknowledged by special ceremonies. These include birth and circumcision for boys (*B'rit milah* or *bris*) and the naming of girls in the synagogue. Adolescence is recognized as coming of age and confirmation of allegiance to the Torah, celebrated by *bar mitzvah* for boys at age 13. *Bat mitzvah* is celebrated for girls at the age of 12 only by non-orthodox congregations (Trepp, 1980). The Jewish focus on *bris* and *bar mitzvah* is comparable to the Irish emphasis on the wake and the Italian focus on wedding (McGoldrick, 1982).

SOCIALIZATION PATTERNS

Hertz and Rosen (1982) noted that Eastern European Jewish families place primary emphasis on four values: centrality of the family, suffering as a shared experience, intellectual achievement and financial success, and verbal expressions of feelings.

The family is central and important as a sacred unit. Historically, procreation was a major function of the family; celibacy was condemned.

Suffering as a shared experience related to the persecution of Jews is viewed historically. It is sometimes assumed that suffering is a basic part of life and may even reinforce a sense of superiority by virtue of this burden of oppression.

This perception of suffering is illustrated by a popular Yiddish saying, *Shver zu zein a yid* ("It's tough to be a Jew") (Hertz & Rosen, 1982, p. 367). The unique experiences of the survivors of the Nazi Holocaust have compounded the sense of suffering for all Jews. Some family members of the survivors appear to doubt their own right to joy and happiness (Epstein, 1979; Rabinowitz, 1976; Mostysser, 1975; Hertz & Rosen, 1982). Thus, hypochondriasis is a commonly observed Jewish syndrome. Although treatment may be sought, there is often a resignation and expectation that life is suffering (Zborowski, 1969).

Intellectual achievement and financial success are extremely important to the Jewish family. A high value was placed on learning in the Jewish *shtetls* since learning is portable and the Jews were constantly on the move. In addition, knowledge earned the student prestige, respect, and status (Dimont, 1978; Hertz & Rosen, 1982). Financial success is an important Jewish family value; however, the act of giving is also important. Today, there is a distinct tendency for Jewish families to be generous and philanthropic (Sklare, 1972; Bloom, 1981).

Verbal expressions of feelings and articulations are readily used by family members, including the children. Jewish families use verbal skills to express pain and anger and are less stoic than some other ethnic groups (Zborowski, 1969). Some popular Jewish expressions are *mazal tov* (good luck, congratulations), *shalom* (peace, hello, or good-bye), and *oy* or *oy vei* (indicates pain or discomfort).

RELIGIOUS BELIEFS AND PRACTICES

Jews believe that the Jewish religion, Judaism, and Jewish people are inseparable. Thus, the denial of religion does not remove the Jew from his or her people. Nonreligious Jews remain committed to the survival of the Jewish people and continue as members of the community of Israel (Trepp, 1980).

It is believed that Judaism originated at Sinai when God entered into a covenant (*B'rit*) with the people of Israel. The Torah, received by Moses and transmitted to Joshua, is the sacred document of that covenant. The Torah, written in Hebrew, presents *mitzvot*, or commandments that govern Jewish life. Rabbis, considered to be authorized by divine mandate, interpreted the Torah in the Talmud.

Jewish affirmation of the covenant is expressed by the following: "The covenant makes us one people linked to the One God. We exist because God exists; we are one because God is One" (Trepp, 1980, p. 3). The Jewish house of worship is called a synagogue, meaning "congregation." It is a house of assembly and "has never been called the House of God, for who can contain God in an earthly abode" (Trepp, 1980, p. 15). The Jewish Sabbath extends from sunset Friday to sunset Saturday. The Torah is read publicly during Sabbath services, as well as on fast and festival days.

The written Torah is sometimes used for protection. Thus, a *mezuzah* is a small scroll containing a portion of the Torah that is affixed to the doorposts in some Jewish homes as guardian of the home. It is positioned diagonally with respect for two great sages of the Middle Ages, one of whom stated that the *mezuzah* should be placed horizontally while the other argued for vertical placement (Trepp, 1980).

Orthodox Jews wear head coverings at all times. The men wear a skull cap or *kippah*. The Yiddish word for this cap is *yarmucha* (or *yarmulka*). It is believed that head covering proclaims that humans are subject to God, whose hand is over all.

Traditionally, Jewish boys are circumcised on the eighth day after birth, a time of complete dependence. Circumcision is a *mitzvah* (commandment) that confirms manliness. Called *B'rit Milah (Bris)*, it is performed by a *mohel*, a religious person knowledgeable in the technique. The *mohel* need not be a rabbi or physician. God-parents are selected, and a celebration usually follows (Trepp, 1980).

Some Jewish High Holy Days

The observance of religious holidays is an important aspect of Jewish-American life-style. In New York City, the public schools and many Jewish places of business close on most of these holidays which include:

- *Rosh Hashanah* (New Year) occurs in the fall. It is celebrated by home visits, greeting cards to family and friends, and festive family meals, including the symbolic apples and honey.
- *Yom Kippur* (Day of Atonement) occurs ten days after Rosh Hashanah. The family usually prays all day in the synagogue. After a family meal, all members over age 13 (unless considered physiologically unsafe) must fast for 24 hours.
- *Chanukah* or *Hanukah* (Feast of Lights) occurs in the winter and lasts 8 days. A candle is lit each night, and gifts are exchanged among family members.
- *Pesach* (Passover) occurs in the spring and lasts for eight days. The family *seder*, a meal consisting of symbolic foods, is eaten, during which time the family recounts the exodus of the Jews from Egypt (Schlesinger, 1974; Trepp, 1980).

CULTURALLY BASED HEALTH BELIEFS AND PRACTICES

The care of the body is a religious obligation of each individual; therefore health care is a *mitzvah* or commandment. It is believed that a body must be healthy to sustain a healthy soul. The Torah indicates that in order to preserve health, a Jew should live prudently and avoid excessive food, drink, sex, sleep, and activity. Cleanliness is also emphasized for health maintenance (Trepp, 1980).

Mikvah is a practice in Judaism consisting of ritual bathing after the menstrual period. This ritual defines women as "unclean" during menstruation. It was found that Jewish women had negative attitudes about menstruation, whether or not they practiced *Mikvah* (Siegel, 1985–1986). The results of a study by Roth-baum and Jackson (1990) found that Jewish women perceived menstruation as making a woman "unclean" to a greater extent than did Catholic or Protestant women.

Historically, Jewish individuals have been interested in the proper care of the body and medical treatment. They tend to be alert to the effects of drugs. Physicians are highly respected in the Jewish culture. Yet Jewish clients will not hesitate to seek a second opinion because they realize that physicians are human and not infallible (Schwartz, 1991; Trepp, 1983).

Health and illness are frequent topics of conversation among Jewish individuals. Jews believe in the importance of prevention. This attitude facilitates client teaching by the nurse. Complaining, moaning, groaning, and crying are acceptable behaviors in the Jewish culture. These behaviors, which may serve as catharsis for the client, may also encourage the family to share in the suffering. Crying out during labor is expected, as it is believed to lessen the pain. Some Jewish clients may be reluctant to take analgesics (considered to be "dope") for fear of addiction (Schwartz, 1991). Visitation of the sick is considered a religious obligation (Schwartz, 1991; Trepp, 1980).

Lipton and Marbach (1984) studied the pain experience of black, Irish, Italian, Jewish, and Puerto Rican patients. They found interethnic similarities for most aspects of the pain experience but also intraethnic variations. Thus culture alone did not determine response to pain.

CULTURAL DIETARY PATTERNS

The laws of Kashrut that govern kosher (*kasher*) dietary practices are contained in the Talmud. According to the laws, animals should be slaughtered by a trained person, a *shohet*, who is supervised by a rabbi. The animal is slaughtered by a deep cut in the throat, which causes unconsciousness. The blood is then allowed to drain out. Kosher meat is soaked in cold water, drained, sprinkled with salt, washed in cold water, and finally cooked (Trepp, 1980).

Food should be accompanied by fluid. A good breakfast is important. Change in diet may be upsetting to the system. Grace is usually said after the meal to thank God for a satisfying meal. Since food is essential to maintain life, the dietary laws may be suspended when life is endangered. Thus hospital clients may eat whatever food is available, including nonkosher foods (Feldman, 1986).

Eden, Kamath, Kohrs, and Olson (1984) studied nutritional locus of control and found that religious and traditional Jewish men and women tended to be more internally oriented than nonreligious/nontraditional Jewish individuals with respect to nutritional behavior. Food plays an important symbolic role during the Jewish Holy Days and festivals. Popular foods during these times include honey, honey cake, carrot tzimmes, holishkes, strudel, potato krugel, cheese blintzes, eggs, matzo, and wine. Kosher wine must be prepared by Jews (Trepp, 1980). Some typical foods are gefilte fish (chopped, seasoned fish), knishes (pastries filled with potatoes or ground meat), kreplach (noodle dough filled with ground meat or cheese), kuchen (many varieties of coffee cake), farfel (noodle dough grated for soup), and bagel (a doughnut-shaped hard yeast roll) (Ensminger, Ensminger, Kolande & Robson, 1983).

Foods considered unclean (*trefah*) include pork, camel, horse, reptiles, birds of prey, and all shellfish and eels. Meat and dairy are not eaten at the same meal, and separate dishes are used for these foods. Therefore, in the hospital, kosher meals should be served on disposable plates (Ensminger et al., 1983). During the eight days of Passover, kosher foods are served. Other foods are avoided, including foods made with leavening or containing grain. Some medications that contain starch or grain alcohol may be refused by the hospitalized Orthodox client (Schwartz, 1991).

MORBIDITY AND MORTALITY

Tay-Sachs disease is a genetic condition most frequently found in Jewish individuals of Eastern European descent. It is a lethal neurodegenerative disorder caused by deficiency of the lysosomal enzyme beta hexosaminidase A (Hex A). The disease results from mutations in the gene (HEXA) and is inherited in autosomal recessive fashion (Strasberg & Clark, 1992; Fernandez, Kaplan, Clow, Hechtman & Scriver, 1992). Carriers are 10 times more frequent in the Ashkenazi Jewish population, and the carrier rate among Jews is about 1 in 31 individuals (Landels, Ellis, Fensom, Greene & Bobrow, 1991; Petersen, Rotter, Cantor, Field, Greenwald, Lim, Roy, Schoenfeld, Lowder & Kaback, 1983). Tay-Sachs is characterized by an accumulation of fatty substances in the brain due to the absence of the fat-metabolizing enzyme. The condition leads to gradual neural and mental degeneration, with death occurring around the age of 3 or 4 years (Schwartz, 1991).

The second most common genetic condition among Jewish Americans is Gaucher disease. Most common in persons of Ashkenazi Jewish ancestry, Gaucher disease is an autosomal-recessive glycolipid storage disease characterized by a deficiency of glucocerebrosidase. The disease is characterized by marked central nervous system impairment, thrombocytopenia, and yellowish pigmentation of the skin. The carrier frequency is about 8.9%, with a birth incidence of 1 in 450 (Beutler, Gelbart, Kuhl, Sorge & West, 1991; Zimram, Gelbart, Westwood, Grabowski & Beutler, 1991).

Inflammatory bowel diseases such as ulcerative colitis and Crohn's disease are more common in European-American-born Jews than in any other white ethnic group. Jewish females develop ulcerative colitis at an earlier age and Crohn's disease at a later age than males. Israeli-born individuals develop both diseases at a young age (Odes, Fraser, & Krawiec 1989).

The risk of colorectal neoplasia was found to be 50% greater in European-born Jews than non-European Jews. The risk for large bowel neoplasia is highest in individuals with a personal history of colorectal neoplasia, inflammatory bowel disease, or past history of cured breast cancer (Odes, Rozea, Ron, Bass, Bat, Keron, Fireman, Shemesh, Krugliak & Fraser, 1992).

Two-thirds of the Jewish population in Israel have been found to be lactose enzyme deficient and thus may display symptoms of milk intolerance, such as nonspecific G.I. pain, contractions, and diarrhea (Schwartz, 1991). Apparently Jews have a low incidence of alcoholism. However, drinking disorders tend to increase with decreased religious affiliation. Some believe that alcoholism increases with acculturation (Mourant, Kopec & Domaniewsks-Sobczak, 1978).

BELIEFS ABOUT DEATH AND DYING

Some Jewish rabbis believe that dying clients should be informed that the condition is serious but not necessarily terminal to preserve hope or allow the clients time to put their affairs in order (Schwartz, 1991). Generally, the Jewish family will not wish to leave dying members alone. During the last minutes of life, all present should remain. It is considered respectful to watch over persons as they pass out of this world (Lamm, 1969).

After death, the eyes and mouth should be closed by a son or the next nearest relative and a sheet drawn over the face. Close relatives may tear their clothing at the moment of confirmed death or later at home prior to the service and the burial. This practice gives vent to momentary anguish and is a sign of grief (Lamm, 1969).

The body should be positioned so that the feet face the doorway. Some Orthodox Jews retain the custom of placing the body (now considered contaminated) on the floor about 20 minutes after death and covering it with a black cloth. The deceased should not be touched or moved when death occurs in the home (Lamm, 1969; Schwartz, 1991). The dead body is considered *tameh*, unclean. Traditionally, before the body is buried, it is washed with lukewarm water and the hair and nails groomed. Then water is symbolically poured over the body under the sheet for the purpose of purification (Trepp, 1980).

Traditionally, mirrors in the house of the deceased are covered in order to acknowledge that the image of God, reflected in the mirrors, has been diminished by the recent death and also to avoid personal vanity at this time of tragedy (Lamm, 1969; Trepp, 1980). Funeral services are usually simple and characterized by the following:

- The coffin should not be ostentatious; traditionally it is made of wood rather than metal.

- Flowers are not usually used. Instead, many Jews prefer contributions to the synagogue, to research, or to charity.

- Traditionally, viewing the body has been considered objectionable theologically and psychologically. However, viewing has become an American custom.

- Ideally the body should be buried within 24 hours after death. Embalming is not practiced in traditional Judaism unless required by state law. If the body is embalmed, the extracted blood is placed in the coffin. Cremation is prohibited (Trepp, 1980).

The seven days of mourning begin immediately after the burial. The mourners (all relatives in the house of the deceased) return home, remove leather shoes, and have a meal of condolence prepared by friends and neighbors. The mourners sit on stools (hence the expression, "sitting *shiva*") for the seven days and do not groom themselves. Their torn garments are worn. Special prayers are said and candles are burned during the period in honor of the deceased (Lamm, 1969; Trepp, 1980). Orthodoxy dictates that the entire period of mourning, which includes five stages (of which *shiva* is third), must last for 12 months (Lamm, 1969).

REFERENCES

Beutler, E., Gelbart, T. Kuhl, W., Sorge, J., & West, C. (1991). Identification of the second common Jewish Gaucher disease mutation makes possible population-based screening for the heterozygous state. *Proceedings, National Academy of Science, United States of America 88*(22), 10544–47.

Bloom, M. (1981). The missing $500,000,000. *Moment, 7,* 30–35.

Bureau of the Census. (1992). *Statistical abstracts.* Washington, DC: Government Printing Office.

Daniels, R. (1990). *Coming to America: A history of immigration and ethnicity in American life.* Princeton, NJ: HarperCollins.

Dimont, M. I. (1978). *The Jews in America: The roots, history, and destiny of American Jews.* New York: Simon & Schuster.

Eden, I., Kamath, S. K., Kohrs, M. B., & Olson, R. E. (1984, November). Perceived control of nutrition behavior: A study of the locus of control theory among healthy subjects. *Journal of American Dietary Association, 84*(11), 1334–39.

Ensminger, A. H., Ensminger, M. E., Kolande, J. E., & Robson, R. K. (1983). *Foods and nutrition encyclopedia.* Clovis, CA: Pegus Press.

Epstein, H. (1979). *Children of the Holocaust.* New York: G. P. Putnam.

Farber, B., Mindel, C. H., & Lazerwitz, B. (1988). The Jewish American family. In C. H. Mindel, R. W. Habenstein & R. Wright, Jr. (Eds.), *Ethnic families in America: Patterns and variations* (3d ed.) (pp. 400–37). New York: Elsevier.

Feldman, D. M. (1986). *Health and medicine in the Jewish tradition.* New York: Crossroad.

Fernandez, M. J., Kaplan, F., Clow, C. L., Hechtman, P., & Scriver, C. R. (1992). Specificity and hexosaminidase assays and DNA analysis for the detection of Tay-Sachs disease gene carriers among Ashkenazic Jews. *Genetic Epidemiology, 9*(3), 169–75.

Gordon, A. I. (1964). *Intermarriage.* Boston: Beacon Press.

Hertz, F. M., & Rosen, E. J. (1982). Jewish families. In M. McGoldrick, J. K. Pearce & J. Giordano (Eds.), *Ethnicity and family therapy* (pp. 364–92). New York: Guilford Press.

Landels, E. C., Ellis, I. H., Fensom, A. H., Green, P. M., & Bobrow, M. (1991). Frequency of the Tay-Sachs disease splice and insertion mutations in the UK Ashkenazi Jewish population. *Journal of Medical Genetics, 28*(3), 177–80.

Lamm, M. (1969). *The Jewish way in death and mourning.* New York: Jonathan David Publishers.

Lipton, J. A., & Marbach, J. J. (1984). Ethnicity and the pain experience. *Social Science Medicine, 19*(12), 1279–98.

McGoldrick, M. (1982). Irish families. In M. McGoldrick, J. P. Pearce, & J. Giordano (Eds.), *Ethnicity and family therapy* (pp. 310–39). New York: Guilford Press.

Mostysser, T. (1975). The weight of the past: Reminiscences of a survivor's child. *Response, 8,* 3–32.

Mourant, A. E., Kopec, A. C., & Domaniewsks-Sobczak, K. (1978). *The genetics of the Jews.* New York: Oxford University Press.

Odes, H. S., Fraser, D., & Krawiec, J. (1989). Inflammatory bowel disease in migrant and native Jewish populations of southern Israel. *Scandinavian Journal of Gastroenterology—Supplement, 170,* 36–38, 50–55.

Odes, H. S., Rozen, P., Ron, E., Bass, D., Bat, L., Keren, S., Fireman, Z., Shemesh, E., Krugliak, P., & Fraser, G. (1992). *Israel Journal of Medical Science, 28*(1 suppl), 21–28.

Petersen, G. M., Rotter, J. I., Cantor, R. M., Field, L. L., Greenwald, S., Lim, J. S., Roy, C., Schoenfeld, V., Lowden, J. A., & Kaback, M. M. (1983). The Tay-Sachs disease gene in North American Jewish population: Geographic variations and origin. *American Journal of Human Genetics, 35*(6), 1258–69.

Rabinowitz, P. (1976). *New lives.* New York: Avon.

Rothbaum, B. O., & Jackson, J. (1990). Religious influence on menstrual attitudes and symptoms. *Women's Health, 16*(1), 63–78.

Schlesinger, B. (1974). The Jewish family and religion. *Journal of Comparative Family Studies, 5*(2), 27–36.

Schwartz, E. A. (1991). Jewish Americans. In J. N. Giger & R. E. Davidhizar (Eds.), *Transcultural nursing: Assessment and intervention* (pp. 491–520). St. Louis: Mosby Year Book.

Siegel, S. J. (1985–1986, Winter). The effect of culture on how women experience menstruation: Jewish women and mikvah. *Women's Health, 10*(4), 63–90.

Sklare, M. (1972). *American Jews.* New York: Random House.

Strasberg, P. M., & Clarke, J. T. (1992). Rapid nonradioactive method for detecting carriers of the major Ashkenazi Jewish Tay-Sachs disease mutations. *Clinical Chemotherapy, 38*(11), 2249–55.

Strole, L., Langner, T., Michael, S., Opler, M. K., & Rennie, T. A. (1962). *Mental health in the Metropolis: Midtown Manhattan study* (Vol. 1). New York: McGraw-Hill.

Trepp, L. (1980). *The complete book of Jewish observance.* New York: Behrman House/ Summit Books.

Zborowski, M. (1969). *People in pain.* San Francisco: Jossey-Bass.

Zimran, A., Gelbart, T., Westwood, B., Grabowski, G. A., & Beutler, E. (1991). High frequency of the Gaucher disease mutation atnucleotide 1226 among Ashkenzi Jews. *American Journal of Human Genetics, 49*(4), 855–59.

13

Korean Americans

Korea is located on a peninsula in East Asia. China and the former Soviet Union border on the north. To the south, the Korean Strait separates Korea from Japan. After the Korean War (1950–1953), close political, economic, and military ties between the United States and South Korea strengthened the American cultural influence in South Korea (Min, 1988; Wagner, 1991).

The climate of Korea varies by region but may be described as having seasonal, windy rainfalls. The average winter temperatures are usually well below freezing, and during the hottest part of the summer, temperatures range between 77 and 80 degrees F (Korean Overseas Information Service, 1979).

POPULATION IN THE UNITED STATES

Koreans comprise the fifth largest Asian group in the United States. Numbering about 800,000 individuals, they represent approximately 0.3% of the American population. The Korean-American population has increased by about 125.3% since the 1980 Census report. The largest number reside in the West (44%), followed by the Northeast (22%), the South (20%), and the lowest number in the Midwest (14%) (Bureau of the Census, 1992). Cities with the largest Korea ancestry population are (in descending order) Los Angeles, New York, Chicago, and Honolulu (Allen & Turner, 1988).

With the exception of "Koreatown" in Los Angeles, Korean immigrants generally have not settled in tightly segregated ethnic communities. Instead, they have settled in and around the urban areas of America, establishing the highest level of suburban residence of all American ethnic groups (Hurh & Chung, 1984; Kim, 1980; Yu, 1983).

IMMIGRATION

The first wave of Korean immigrants to America began in 1903 when about 7,000 men came to Hawaii to work on sugar plantations (Kim, 1980). In the 1950s, during and after the Korean War, many Korean women came to America as war brides, married to U.S. servicemen. Intermarriages between Korean women and American men and adoptions of Korean orphans by American citizens are practices that continue today. Most Korean Americans are either post–Korean War immigrants or their descendants. Korean Americans show the highest rate of naturalization of all Asian-American groups (Daniels, 1990; Min, 1988; Ryu, 1977).

COMMUNICATION

Most Korean Americans speak some English. Many display a close comfort zone with family (especially parents and children) but may be distant with other people. Nonverbal behavior such as moving the body or turning the head away from another person may indicate an invasion of the Korean American's personal comfort zone (Watson, 1970).

SOCIOECONOMIC STATUS

Korean Americans exhibit a high rate of self-employment. Many Korean Americans work in small family-owned enterprises such as fruit and vegetable stands, grocery stores, dry cleaners, restaurants, and nail care salons. Some first- and second-generation Korean Americans work long hours in family businesses, which may make them prone to physical and emotional stress. Others are involved in the wholesale and retail trade of imported Korean items (Daniels, 1990; Min, 1988). Because of an increase in nursing education for women in Korea and the nursing shortage in America, many Korean women immigrants are nurses (Bullough & Bullough, 1982; Kim, 1984).

Most Korean-American families tend to place high emphasis on education as essential to upward social mobility. Sometimes parental pressure for high scholastic achievement may be stressful for Korean-American children (Butterfield, 1990; Min, 1988). Many recent Korean immigrants are of high social class with a heavy concentration of educated professionals and technicians (Min, 1988).

CHIEF COMPLAINT

Korean-American clients' descriptions of pain may vary from stoic to expressive. Some Korean Americans have a high pain tolerance level (Kim, 1989).

Many value self-control, which places responsibility for behavior on forces within the individual. Some Korean Americans choose to suppress their emotions in public. For example, joy is not usually expressed by shouting, jumping up and down, dancing, or embracing but most often in a quiet manner (Kim, 1989). If the client appears reserved, the health professional should note nonverbal signs of distress, such as hyperactivity and unusual facial expressions. Physiological indicators of discomfort include elevated blood pressure, increased pulse and heart rates, and diaphoresis.

FAMILY

Confucianism, the traditional philosophy of Korean thought and behavior, has influenced the relationships among members of Korean families (Korean Overseas Information Service, 1979). Confucian teachings emphasize patriarchy, filial piety, and educational achievement (Min, 1988). The traditional Korean family has the following characteristics:

- *Patriarchy.* The father is the head of the household, authority, primary breadwinner, and decision maker in the family.
- *Extended structure.* In addition to the parents and their children, the family might include other relatives, such as in-laws, uncles, aunts, cousins, grandparents, and grandchildren, living together or in close proximity.
- *Continuity.* In a patrilineal rule of descent, the oldest son is the father's heir. The family's name and lineage are passed down through the male members (Kim, 1989).
- *Inclusiveness.* A strong kinship organization is based on patrilocal rule of residence and genealogical records (Kim, 1989).
- *Authority.* The father has unchallengeable authority over his wife and the children, the elders control the younger members, and the males dominate the females (Kim, 1989).
- *Asexuality.* The father-son relationship is more important than the husband-wife relationship. Arranged marriage is a basic manifestation of asexuality in Korean kinship (Kim, 1989; Min, 1988).
- *Filial piety (hyo'song).* This special obligation requires that the eldest son remain with his parents after his marriage in order to ensure them care and financial support. Filial piety is extended even after death through ancestor worship (Min, 1988).
- The role of women was directed by the Confucian philosophy that a female must conform to a Rule of Three Following. She must follow her father as a child, her husband as an adult, and her son when she is old (Kim, 1989; Shon & Ja, 1982).

Traditional Marriage Practices

Many marriages have been arranged among families by the elders (Min, 1988). Girls often are married at about age 15, while boys are generally three to four years younger (Korean Overseas Information Service, 1979).

A woman's charm, beauty, and sex appeal usually are not important qualifications of a suitable bride. Instead, selection criteria include physical characteristics, such as long and narrow eyebrows, a flat forehead with smoothly curved eyebrows, broad hips with a large stomach, and light and bright skin color (Lee, 1981, pp. 370–71). These characteristics are believed conducive to bearing children, especially sons (Kim, 1989).

Ideally, traditional Korean couples remain aloof from each other, symbolic of asexuality. Sexual pleasure between husband and wife is less important than bearing a male heir. They seldom display affection in public, especially in the presence of their respected parents and elders (Kim, 1989).

Modern Families

Most second-generation Korean-Americans, between 35 and 45 years of age, tend to be strongly influenced by American mainstream family practices. Generally, modern Korean marriages are no longer arranged by families, and relationships between husband and wife are more egalitarian (Min, 1988).

For many second-generation Korean-American families to maintain a successful small business, both husband and wife must work together. A wife's help in the store (usually as the cashier) is essential to the success of the business, affording her an economic role equal to that of her husband in the family (Min, 1988). Nevertheless, the husband is usually the family leader and major decision maker in the family. The mother's level of education is the most important factor in determining her decision-making power in the family relative to her husband, especially in child-rearing matters (Jook & Kyong-dong, 1977). Still, Korean immigrant couples tend to be less egalitarian than the average American couple with respect to decision making (Min, 1988).

A low divorce rate, low percentage of female-headed households, and high percentage of couple families foster a high degree of family stability among Korean immigrants (Min, 1988; Tienda & Angel, 1982).

ELDERLY

Because Confucian ideology places emphasis on age, the elderly are usually highly respected and viewed as authorities by the family. In the event of illness, the elder's son and his wife assume responsibility for the parents' health care (Min, 1988).

CHILD REARING

Traditional parents may treat unmarried individuals as children regardless of age. Boys and girls part their hair in the middle and wear it in two braids to signify that they are minors. Traditionally boys and girls are separated at the age of seven, at which time they attend separate schools and engage in different

activities (Korean Overseas Information Service, 1979). Traditional infant ceremonies include an elaborate banquet held on the hundredth day after birth if
the child is a first son, and a banquet held on a baby's first birthday, when the
child's future is predicted depending on which symbolic item placed before the
child attracts his or her attention first (Korean Overseas Information Service,
1979).

Modern Practices

Korean Americans average about two or three children per family (Min,
1988). Some parents establish extremely close ties with their infants and children, who receive such constant attention that some Americans view this behavior as overindulgence (Butterfield, 1990).

Generally, second-generation Korean parents tend to be less authoritarian than
first-generation parents. Also, they are not likely to assign the first son authority
over his younger brothers and sisters (Min, 1988).

Since many Korean-American women may be active participants in family-
owned businesses, as well as the general labor force, their children may be
taught to share the household duties. However, household responsibilities tend
to reflect gender role socialization. For example, boys rarely do kitchen duties
(Min, 1988).

Discipline

Korean-American children are taught to respect their parents and other elders
(Shon & Ja, 1982). They are expected to use expressions and gestures when
interacting with adults that are different from those used with their peers (Min,
1988). Korean-American parents tend to use punishment more often than American parents and give monetary rewards for good behavior less often than American parents (Min, 1988).

SOCIALIZATION PATTERNS

Most Korean Americans are either post–Korean War immigrants or their descendants. Many older clients may be first-generation Korean Americans. Because of their exposure to Western values and beliefs before migration, many
individuals from South Korea on all generational levels have readily accepted
many American cultural practices (Min, 1988). The high rate of Korean naturalization may imply an inclination to adapt and a willingness to integrate into
the American cultural system. Therefore, this client and family could most likely
exhibit health behaviors that are similar to those of mainstream Americans (Ryu,
1977; Min, 1988).

Some Korean Americans attempt to maintain harmony and avoid conflict in
social interactions. Because second- and third-generation Korean Americans

tend to be highly acculturated, their behavior during social interactions may be similar to those of the average American (Min, 1988).

Korean Americans typically respect authority and may use gestures or expressions that convey respect: bowing the head when addressing the professional, showing agreement, and not asking questions even when he or she does not understand information or instructions. Some Korean-American individuals feel that asking a question of an authority is disrespectful because it indicates that the professional initially failed to make the information clear. Rather than ask the Korean-American client, "Do you understand?" the health care provider should instead ask the client to repeat the information to verify that it was understood (Chang, 1981; Kim, 1989).

Some Korean-American women tend to display more behavioral restraints and are more reserved than Korean-American men. Exposure of body parts may cause embarrassment especially to Korean-American women clients. The health provider should respect a client's modesty and need for privacy during care. Many may refrain from overt expressions of emotion; families may display limited overt expressions such as hugging and kissing. Some first-generation Korean Americans may display asexual behavior and control of emotions in public (Kim, 1989).

RELIGIOUS BELIEFS AND PRACTICES

Three religious and philosophical traditions in Korean culture—Confucianism, Buddhism, and Taoism—have significantly shaped Korean-American attitudes about life and death, self-care, and social interactions.

Confucianism

This philosophy of government and guide to moral conduct as modified in Korea is called neo-Confucianism. Ancestor worship, an integral part of Confucianism, is based on the belief that the dead remain as they were at death and retain the same requirements for shelter, clothing, and food. Therefore, graves are maintained and clothing and food are offered at neo-Confucian ancestor worship rites. A religious specialist (*mudang*) usually performs the rites, and the spirits act through his or her body. *Mudangs* were usually women (Suk-jay, Janelli & Janelli, 1988; Moon, 1974).

Buddhism

Religious principles developed from the teachings of Guatama Buddha of India. Buddhism emphasizes that enlightenment is attained through intuitive understanding and experienced through meditation. Koreans adapted Buddhism and integrated a number of their deities into Buddhist rituals. Ancestor worship is also an integral part of Korean Buddhist practices (Suk-jay, Janelli & Janelli, 1988).

Taoism

This practice, based on the philosophy of Lao Tzu (or Laotse), emphasizes the mystical aspects of human nature. It focuses on attaining the optimal state of well-being, which is in harmony with cosmological and natural spheres (Kleinman & Lin, 1981).

Modern Korean-American Religious Practices

Christian values and beliefs became more prominent in South Korea during and after the Korean War. Therefore, unlike other Asians, recent Korean immigrants to the United States are predominantly Christians, usually Protestants. Yet Protestantism remains a minority religion in Korea because Protestants and other Christians, who are more familiar with American beliefs and values, tend to migrate (Kim, 1980; Min, 1988).

Protestant beliefs focus on the Trinity: God, the Father; God, the Son (Jesus); and God, the Holy Spirit. The Bible (Old and New Testaments) is the document of authority, but each individual assumes responsibility for his or her religious life. Preaching and the singing of hymns are significant methods of worship. Fasting and meditation are often practiced. Protestants usually worship on Sunday.

Protestant religious observances include baptism, confirmation, marriage, and funeral rites (Prebish, 1987; Filiault, 1991; Jones, 1994).

Some Protestant Korean Americans believe that healing depends on medical intervention directed by God and prefer to rely on divine intervention rather than herbs, potions, or rituals (Prebish, 1987). The Korean-American client may need periods alone or with family members to pray, meditate, affirm wellness, or sing hymns. Sometimes the health professional may pray or sing hymns with this client. Singing of hymns could be emotionally therapeutic to a client whose prognosis is poor or to a comatose client. Although comatose clients do not respond, auditory stimulation such as music and the human voice is a recommended therapeutic measure (Beare & Myers, 1990).

CULTURALLY BASED HEALTH BELIEFS AND PRACTICES

Many Korean Americans believe in a holistic concept of health and view health and illness as an integration of biological, social, psychological, and emotional aspects of the human. This holistic concept also emphasizes the inseparable nature of mind and body. Therefore, some believe that health professionals should consider the interactions of mental and physical symptoms, as well as address the social implications of the client's condition (Do, 1988).

Some Korean Americans believe in concepts of balance between humans and the universe, yin and yang, hot and cold. The yin state is associated with symptoms of "internal cold" and reduced body function, whereas symptoms of the yang state indicate a generalized hyperactivity with external manifestations such as a "warm" sensation and/or an elevated temperature (Tien-Hyatt, 1987). (A detailed discussion of yin and yang is contained in Chapter 3 on Chinese Americans).

Korean-American folk health practices tend to vary from the use of *mudang* or shamans (mediums), herbalists, and acupuncturists to American mainstream medical methods (Kraut, 1990). Some traditional Korean-American clients who practice ancestor worship may seek advice or assistance from spirits through a shaman or medium. Often this practice does not replace or influence the medical therapeutic regime (Moon, 1974).

The practice of acupuncture is based on the concept of vital energy forces (negative yin and positive yang) within the body and the universe. These forces circulate through the body along meridians similar to blood, lymph, and nerves. Acupuncture is a method of preventing and treating pain and disease by the skilled insertion of special needles into designated points (1,000 known points) on the skin at various depths and angles for varying lengths of time. Acupuncture is superior to general anesthetics for some surgical procedures because the client remains awake and alert, and there are no postanesthesia blood pressure and respiratory complications (Beare & Myers, 1990; Miller & Keane, 1987).

Ginseng or ginseng root (often called the root of life) may be used by some Korean Americans as a rejuvenator for pregnant women, athletes, older persons, or anyone in a weakened condition. Ginseng is also believed to be an aphrodisiac (Andrews, 1989). The health professional should be alert to adverse reactions associated with the long-term use of ginseng, such as nervousness, insomnia, edema, or irregularities in blood glucose levels (Ginseng, 1980; Siegel, 1979).

Middle-class Korean Americans tend to share health-related values and practices with the American mainstream culture, although those who follow Western health methods often retain some traditional remedies for selected illnesses and practice them concurrently or consecutively with Western health care (Chang, 1981; Do, 1988; Kraut, 1990).

CULTURAL DIETARY PATTERNS

Rice is the staple food of the Korean diet. In order to add nutrients, white rice is often boiled with barley, millet, and red beans. Rice cakes are favorites. Fish (raw, steamed, salted, or dried) and soybean products (soy sauce, bean curd or tofu, soy milk) are major sources of dietary protein. Soups containing fish, beef, or seaweed are served frequently.

Korean-American diets include fresh fruits and vegetables. Vegetables are lightly cooked to preserve crispness and nutrients and highly seasoned with red and black pepper, garlic, and soy sauce. Food is preferred chopped in small pieces that are easy to manage with chopsticks. Barley water, a favorite beverage, usually accompanies every meal, served cold in the summer and warm in the winter (Burtis, Davis & Martin, 1989; Korean Overseas Information Service, 1979). A popular dish is *kimchi*, prepared with chopped vegetables that are highly seasoned, salted, and fermented for one to three months. Some variety of *kimchi* is usually served at each meal. Because *kimchi* is not readily available in the United States, a Mexican salsa may be an acceptable substitute. Beef, heavily marinated with sugar to produce a crisp coating, is also a favorite (Burtis, Davis & Martin, 1989).

Strict Buddhists are vegetarians; they avoid eating the flesh of any animal except fish. The sin is not in the eating but rather in the killing. Fish are not thought of as killed; rather, they are removed from the sea. Many Buddhists refrain from eggs, milk, and intoxicating beverages (Ensminger, Ensminger, Kolande & Robson, 1983).

Korean Americans usually consume more fruits and vegetables than meats. The disadvantages of a low protein or a vegetarian diet are most significant during periods of high body protein requirement, such as infancy, growth, stress, surgery, and illness. Inadequate dietary protein could delay healing, compromise the immune system, or slow a child's growth rate (Burtis, Davis & Martin, 1989).

Koreans tend to use seasonings that are high in sodium. If sodium is restricted (e.g., cardiovascular conditions), the health professional may suggest methods of preparing foods with tasty herbal and garlic spices instead of salt and monosodium glutamate. Some meats are heavily marinated with sugar. When sugar intake must be limited (e.g., diabetes or obesity), a sugar substitute may be used in the preparation of beef to achieve a crispy coating. Due to the high acculturation of Korean Americans, many individuals have adopted American dietary habits, and consequently, obesity among Korean Americans is not uncommon (Freimer, Echenberg & Kretchmer, 1983).

MORBIDITY AND MORTALITY

Lactose enzyme deficiency is found in about 90% of Korean-American adults. Individuals with this condition are unable to digest the lactose in milk and many dairy products (Chang, 1981). Symptoms of lactose intolerance include gastrointestinal upset, cramping, and diarrhea. If lactose intolerance is a problem, the client and family should be informed about lactose-free products on the market. Cheese aged over 60 days may be eaten because lactose is converted to lactic acid during the aging process (Chang, 1981).

One potentially life-threatening illness that soldiers faced during the Korean War and still exists today is Korean hemorrhagic fever (Gill, 1991). Hemorrhagic fever with renal syndrome (HFRS) is characterized by fever, headache, fatigue, abdominal pain, renal dysfunction, and various hemorrhagic manifestations. A lethal form of the disease occurs in Korea, and a milder, nonlethal form is found in Europe. HFRS is endemic in a belt from Norway in the west, through Sweden, Finland, the former Soviet Union, China, Korea to Japan in the east. The clinical severity varies throughout this belt. The disease is caused by hantaviruses spread by rodents and transmitted to humans via aerosol from rodent urine, saliva, and feces (Niklasson, 1992).

BELIEFS ABOUT DEATH AND DYING

Christian Korean Americans tend to believe that illness and death are determined by fate, which God has destined, and that one must go peacefully to the final destination. Some Korean-American Protestants believe that group prayers and hymns foster a peaceful death or transition to another life (Tien-Hyatt, 1987).

PHYSICAL ASSESSMENT

Generally, Korean Americans tend to be shorter than the average American individual (Overfield, 1985). American mainstream growth and development standards may be inappropriate to use for the physical assessment of some Korean-American children (Chang, 1981).

Some Korean Americans tend to have small noses (Chang, 1981). This factor may be significant if the client requires nasal oxygen or the insertion of nasogastric tubes.

The epicanthic fold of the eyelids is a vertical fold found at the inner corners of the eyes, causing the eyes to appear far apart. This is a normal finding among Korean Americans (Chang, 1981; Miller & Keane, 1987).

Mongolian spots, bluish discolorations sometimes found on the lower back, are normal for Korean-American individuals (Chang, 1981).

REFERENCES

Allen, J. P., & Turner, E. J. (1988). *We the people: Atlas of American ethnic diversity.* New York: Macmillan.

Andrews, M. M. (1989). Culture and nutrition. In J. S. Boyle & M. M. Andrews (Eds.), *Transcultural concepts in nursing care* (pp. 333–35). Glenview, IL: Scott, Foresman/Little, Brown.

Beare, P. G., & Myers, J. L. (1990). *Principles and practice of adult health nursing.* St. Louis: C. V. Mosby Co.

Bullough, B., & Bullough, V. (1982). *Nursing in the community.* St. Louis: C. V. Mosby Co.

Bureau of the Census. (1991). *1990 counts on specific racial groups.* Washington, DC: Government Printing Office.

Burtis, G., Davis, J., & Martin, S. (1989). *Applied nutrition and diet therapy.* Philadelphia: W. B. Saunders Company.

Butterfield, F. (1990, January). Why they excel: What we can learn from our Asian

American students who are winning top honors and jobs. *Social Issues Resources Series, 4*(2), 4–6.

Chang, B. (1981). Asian-American patient care. In G. Henderson & M. Primeaux (Eds.), *Transcultural health care* (pp. 255–78). Menlo Park, CA: Addison-Wesley.

Chrisman, N. J., & Kleinman, A. (1980). Health beliefs and practices. In S. Thernstrom (Ed.), *Harvard encyclopedia of American ethnic groups* (pp. 452–61). Cambridge, MA: Belknap Press of Harvard University Press.

Daniels, R. (1990). *Coming to America: A history of immigration and ethnicity in American life.* Princeton, NJ: HarperCollins.

Do, H. K. (1988). *Health and illness beliefs and practices of Korean Americans.* Unpublished doctoral dissertation, Boston University.

Ensminger, A. H., Ensminger, M. E., Kolande, J. E., & Robson, R. K. (1983). Religions and diets. In *Foods and nutrition encyclopedia* (Vol. 2) (pp. 1914–20). Clovis, CA: Pegus Press.

Filiault, P. (1991, October). Interview.

Freimer, N., Echenberg, D., & Kretchmer, N. (1983). Cultural variation: Nutritional and clinical implications. *Western Journal of Medicine, 139*(6), 928–32.

Gill, P. M. (1991). Korean hemorrhagic fever: Nursing care critical to recovery. *Military Medicine, 156*(3), 131–34.

Ginseng. (1980). *Medical Letter Drugs Therapy, 22*(17), 72.

Hurh, W. M., & Chung, K. K. (1984). *Korean immigrants in North America: Structural analysis of ethnic confinement and adhesive adaptation.* Madison: Fairleigh Dickinson University Press.

Jook, L. K., & Kyong-dong, K. (1977). A cultural interpretation of the effects of mother's employment status on parental decision making role patterns in the Korean family. *Journal of Comparative Family Studies, 8*(1).

Jones, R. (1994, August). Interview with author.

Kim, C. S. (1989). Attribute of ''asexuality'' in Korean kinship and sundered Koreans during the Korean War. *Journal of Comparative Family Studies, 20*(3), 309–25.

Kim, H. (1980). Koreans. In S. Thernstrom (Ed.), *The Harvard encyclopedia of American ethnic groups* (pp. 601–6). Cambridge: Belknap Press of Harvard University Press.

Kim, S. (1984, Fall). The role of women in health care in Korea's social transition. *Image: The Journal of Nursing Scholarship, 16*(4), pp. 99–101.

Kleinman, A., & Lin, T. Y. (1981). *Normal and abnormal behavior in Chinese culture.* Boston: Reidel Publishing Co.

Korean Overseas Information Service. (1979). *A Handbook of Korea.* Seoul, Korea: Ministry of Culture and Information.

Kraut, A. M. (1990). Healers and strangers: Immigrant attitudes toward the physician in America—A relationship in historical perspective. *JAMA, 263*(13), pp. 1807–11.

Lee, K. (1981). *Structure of the Korean thought pattern.* Seoul: Munri-sa.

Miller, B. F., & Keane, C. B. (1987). *Encyclopedia and dictionary of medicine, nursing, and allied health.* Philadelphia: W. B. Saunders.

Min, P. G. (1988). The Korean American family. In C. H. Mindel, R. W. Haberstein & R. Wright, Jr. (1988), *Ethnic families in America: Patterns and variations* (3d ed.). New York: Elsevier.

Moon, S. G. (1974). Ancestor worship in Korea: Tradition and transition. *Journal of Comparative Family Studies, 5*(2), 71–87.

Niklasson, B. S. (1992). Hemorrhagic fever with renal syndrome, viriological and epidemiological aspects. *Pediatric Nephrology, 6*(2), 201–4.

Overfield, T. (1985). *Biological variations in health and illness: Race, age and sex differences.* Reading, MA: Addison-Wesley.

Prebish, C. S. (1987). Protestantism. In M. Eliade (Ed.), *The encyclopedia of religion* (Vol. 12) (pp. 23–38). New York: Macmillan.

Ryu, J. P. (1977). Koreans in America: A demographic analysis. In Hyung-chan kim (Ed.), *The Korean diaspora: Historical and sociological studies of Korean immigration and assimilation in North America* (pp. 205–28). Santa Barbara, CA: ABC-Clio.

Shon, S. P., & Ja, D. Y. (1982). Asian families. In M. McGoldrick, J. E. Pearce & J. Giordano (Eds.), *Ethnicity and family therapy* (pp. 208–28). New York: Guilford Press.

Siegel, R. K. (1979). Ginseng abuse syndrome: Problems with the panacea. *JAMA, 24*(15), 614.

Suk-jay, Y., Janelli, R. L., & Janelli, D. Y. (1987). Korean religion. In M. Eliade (Ed.), *The encyclopedia of religion* (Vol. 8) (pp. 367–76). New York: Macmillan.

Tienda, M., & Angel, R. (1982). Headship and household comparison among blacks, Hispanics and other whites. *Social Forces, 61*, 508–31.

Tien-Hyatt, Juliet L. (1987). Keying in on the unique care needs of Asian clients. *Nursing and Health Care, 8*(5), 268–71.

Wagner, E. W. (1990). Korea. In *Encyclopedia Americana: International edition* (pp. 543–45). Danbury, CT: International Headquarters.

Watson, O. M. (1970). *Proxemic behavior; A cross-cultural study.* The Hague, Netherlands: Mouton.

Yu, Eui-young. (1983). Korean communities in America: Past, present, and future. *Amerasia Journal, 19*, 23–52.

14

Mexican Americans

Mexico (or the United Mexican States) is located in the southern part of North America. Mexico, consisting of 31 states and a federal district, is the third largest nation in Latin America, after Brazil and Argentina. On the southeast, Mexico shares borders with Guatemala and Belize in Central America. The Pacific Ocean and the Gulf of California lie to the west, and the Gulf of Mexico and the Caribbean Sea to the east of Mexico.

Mexico's land area consists largely of hills and mountainous terrains with lower valleys and coastal areas, and the climate varies by region. The coastal sections usually experience warm to hot temperatures most of the year, while temperatures in the mountains and highlands are cool to cold year round. The most favorable climate, described as temperate, is found in the highland valleys (Rudolph, 1985).

POPULATION IN THE UNITED STATES

There are about 13.5 million Mexican Americans in the United States, which constitutes 5.4% of the total U.S. population. Mexican Americans are the second largest minority group in this country, representing about 60% of the total Hispanic population. The largest numbers reside in the West (57%), followed by the South (33%), with the smallest populations in the Midwest (9%) and the Northeast (1%) (Bureau of the Census, 1992). About 86% of Mexican Americans reside in the five southwestern states of California, Texas, Arizona, Colorado, and New Mexico (Becerra, 1988). The city of Los Angeles has the highest concentration of Mexican Americans, followed by San Antonio and Houston, Texas (Allen & Turner, 1988).

Many Mexican Americans reside in crowded Hispanic sections. This practice of voluntary segregation enhances group identification. Mexican Americans have been more persistent than many other ethnic groups in maintaining their language, culture, and traditions (Reinert, 1986).

IMMIGRATION

Between 1880 and 1910, during the years of rapid economic development in the United States, Mexicans migrated to assume low-wage jobs in mining, railroad construction, and agriculture. In the early 1900s there was a major wave of immigrants escaping the violence of the Mexican Revolution of 1910. In the 1960s, young Mexican-American activists started the Chicano movement, which focused on overcoming problems of limited educational opportunities, high unemployment rate, low wages, and general low socioeconomic status of Mexican Americans. The term *Chicano* was used to denote a politically alert and active American of Mexican descent (Becerra, 1988).

Most Mexicans are *mestizos*, of mixed Spanish and Indian descent (Falicov, 1982; Rudolph, 1985). Mexican Americans refer to themselves in different ways according to their varied histories—for example, Chicano, Tejano, Californio, Mexican American, or Spanish American (Daniels, 1990).

Due to the proximity of Mexico to the United States, there has been continuous interaction and migration between the two countries. Many Mexicans continue to enter the United States in search of improved economic opportunities. Some individuals arrive in the United States with the appropriate documents, some overstay their visa arrangement and become undocumented, and yet others enter as undocumented aliens. The number of undocumented aliens of Mexican descent is difficult to determine. Mexican Americans suffer discrimination in housing, education, and employment (Becerra, 1988; Falicov, 1982; Kuipers, 1991).

COMMUNICATION

Most Mexican Americans speak Spanish, the third most commonly spoken language in the world (Monrroy, 1983). Translations of some Spanish terms are presented at the end of Chapter 4, on Cuban Americans.

Mexican Americans are generally quite tactile. For example, a pat on a child's head signifies admiration. If the family believes in the evil eye, touching will dispel the evil. Some may prefer a close personal space zone during an interview. Mexican Americans take pride in their art of verbal expression, which may be elaborate and dramatic and often indirect (Falicov, 1982; Murillo, 1978).

SOCIOECONOMIC STATUS

Although some Mexican Americans are well educated, most are not. In 1986 the total percentage of Mexican Americans who had completed high school or higher was 38% (Bureau of the Census, 1988). As Mexicans have learned English and begun to speak it more fluently, the level of education has increased. A major issue is the lack of American citizenship, which serves as a barrier to gaining education, skills, stable jobs, decent living conditions, and government benefits. Lower socioeconomic status Mexican families tend to resist acculturation and show stronger ethnic identification than Mexican families of higher socioeconomic status (Kuipers, 1991; Valdez, 1980).

CHIEF COMPLAINT

In order to avoid any show of weakness, a macho male may be stoic and bear his discomfort for an extended period of time. Women and children are permitted to be more expressive and usually describe their symptoms and pain or discomfort more readily (Bullough & Bullough, 1982; Kuipers, 1991).

Although Mexican Americans' self-report of pain may be higher than that of other cultural groups (African Americans and Caucasians), their endurance may be greater. This ability to endure pain is considered admirable, courageous, and self-sacrificing. Many Mexican Americans accept pain as an expected and necessary aspect of human life. Some perceive pain and suffering as characteristic of the fate of humans on earth. Thus, some Mexican Americans are less likely than Caucasian groups to state medical or scientific reasons as the cause of pain because they view pain and suffering as punishment (castigo) for sins and manifested by family misfortune such as hunger, thirst, and/or disease (Villarruel & de Montellano, 1992).

FAMILY

Traditional Family

Although practices vary among individual families, they are derived from traditional beliefs and practices of working-class individuals in rural and semirural areas of Mexico. Two concepts of traditional family structure have existed: nuclear and extended (Murillo, 1978).

The family is the major support system and has been more important than each individual member. The system has been patriarchal, patrilocal, and patrilineal. In the patriarchal model, the father has been the powerful, authoritative head of the household and the major decision maker (Becerra, 1988; Falicov, 1982). In the patrilocal family, the young married couple lives with the husband's family. A good relationship between the daughter-in-law and the mother-in-law is crucial to the success of the marriage (Falicov, 1982). The patrilineal factor acknowledges the father's family as more important than the mother's family (Murillo, 1978).

Machismo or *muy hombre* means "manliness" or "virility." Machismo depicts men as aggressive, sexually experienced, courageous, generous, and protective of their women. The *macho*, exemplifying male dominance, demands allegiance and obedience from his wife and children (Becerra, 1988; Falicov, 1982). Although many men have had to leave their families in order to find work, during which time their wives became heads of the household, the ideology of patriarchy has persisted (Griswold del Castillo, 1984).

Ideally females have been humble, submissive, virtuous, and devoted to their children. The relationship between mother and daughter has been particularly close (Murillo, 1978). There has been a hierarchical order of rigid gender and age grading, with females subordinate to males and the younger subordinate to the older (Falicov, 1982).

Modern Family

Mexican Americans appear to have more cohesive family support than many other ethnic groups (Griswold del Castillo, 1984). Mexican-American men are more likely than any other cultural group to take on a single-parent role, and they tend to take over the household tasks more often when no woman is present (Becerra, 1988).

Modern families are generally nuclear and are thus less likely to have extended kin living in the same household, although they usually reside nearby. There appears to be increasing social and economic mobility of Mexican-American families, manifested by the increasing number of Mexican Americans in professional and managerial positions (Becerra, 1988). Autonomy and individual achievement are being encouraged in some families, as evidenced by the increasing numbers of college and university students of Mexican descent (Becerra, 1988; Falicov, 1982). Some modern Mexican-American families are moving toward an egalitarian husband-wife relationship (Becerra, 1988).

CHILD REARING

Mexican-American families usually have a large number of children. The relationship between parents and children is considered more important than the marital relationship (Falicov, 1982).

The results of a study by McKenzie, Sallis, Nader, Broyles & Nelson (1992) suggested that Mexican-American children tend to spend more time in the presence of adults, play with fewer action toys, and thus were found to be less physically active than Anglo children. Extended family members such as grandparents, uncles, aunts, and godparents often provide nurturance and support for the young, as well as some control over adolescents (Falicov, 1982).

Godparents: The *Compadrazo* System

Godparents are an extension of the family. The custom of maintaining god-parents establishes two important relationships: between the *padrinos y ahijados* (godparents and their godchildren) and the formal relationship between parents and godparents who become *compadres* (coparents). Godparents may or may not be chosen from among members of the extended family. Sometimes individuals of a higher socioeconomic status than the family are selected in order to extend the child's economic resources. Godparents chosen at baptism usually assume responsibility throughout the child's life. Godparents chosen at marriage contribute to the wedding expenses and in theory may mediate in the couple's quarrels (Falicov, 1982; Kuipers, 1991). Baptism and marriage are the most important life cycle rituals for Mexican Americans (Falicov, 1982).

Discipline

The Mexican-American father disciplines and controls his children. He is usually playful and affectionate toward young children but a firm disciplinarian with his children after puberty. At this time, siblings are segregated by gender; boys socialize strictly with boys and girls with girls. Common methods of dis-cipline within the family are scolding, shaming or belittling, deception, promises, and threats (Falicov, 1982).

Children are expected to help with all work around the house. Although many Mexican-American families emphasize good behavior and obedience to their children, the concepts of achievement and attainment of self-reliance are not generally stressed. Education in Anglo schools has been unpopular because it was believed to cause a breakdown of family unity (Falicov, 1982; Murillo, 1978).

SOCIALIZATION PATTERNS

Mexican Americans often have the following characteristics:

- Machismo and male dominance
- Female submissiveness
- Generational interdependence
- Strong sense of family loyalty
- Fatalism
- Honesty and dignity
- Personalism (a focus on relationships rather than tasks) (Levine & Padilla, 1980)

Many Mexican Americans appear highly sensual. They love to touch, feel, and smell. They like sounds, including lively music, bright colors, activity, and spicy foods. To the Mexican American, the Anglo may appear distant, cold, and insensitive.

Mexican Americans are sometimes characterized as having a present time orientation. For example, the Mexican custom of siesta may represent a priority of rest at present over work for future output (Kuipers, 1991). For the Mexican, time is not based on the Anglo concept of "time is money." Instead responsibility focuses on other values, such as meeting the needs of family and friends. This priority of values may cause a Mexican American to arrive late for an appointment. This present time orientation may serve as a barrier to integration into mainstream American culture and may even restrain some Mexican Americans from upward social and economic mobility (Kuipers, 1991; Murillo, 1978).

A cultural Indian concept of limited good proposed that there is only so much good in the world and only so much good that can be achieved in a lifetime. Mexican Americans are somewhat likely to believe in an external locus of control. This could promote a fatalistic outlook and foster the belief that an individual is at the mercy of the environment (Kuipers, 1991; Murillo, 1978).

RELIGIOUS BELIEFS AND PRACTICES

Mexican Americans are predominantly Roman Catholic (Daniels, 1990; Kuipers, 1991). Traditional native Mexican-American beliefs hold that fate is determined by the gods, and there is a reciprocal relationship between humans and the gods. This concept is evident in their beliefs about the body, pain, health, and illness (Villarruel & de Montellano, 1992).

Some Mexican Americans may believe that the body contains multiple souls, divine forces, or animistic centers. One such animistic force is known as *tonalli*. The *tonalli* connects humans to cosmic agents, causing open boundaries that facilitate interaction between humans, nature, and the supernatural. The *tonalli*, believed to be located at the top of one's head, can determine a person's temperament, future behavior, and fate (Villarruel & de Montellano, 1992).

CULTURALLY BASED HEALTH BELIEFS AND PRACTICES

Many Mexican Americans view health as a harmonious relationship between social and spiritual realms (Lawson, 1990). Mexican-American traditional folk medicine and practices tend to persist in the United States as an alternative to scientific medicine for the treatment of minor health problems, psychosocial problems, and chronic conditions that persist in spite of treatment by mainstream health professionals (Reinert, 1986). Some traditional health beliefs that originated with Hippocrates were brought to Mexico by the *conquistadores* (Spanish conquerors). For example, Hippocrates' humoral pathology was based on the belief that the body is composed of four humors—blood, phlegm, black bile, and yellow bile—all associated with specific characteristics: blood is related to hot and wet, phlegm to cold and wet, black bile to cold and dry, and yellow bile to hot and dry. Organs of the body were categorized in terms of these humors; for example, the heart was considered to be hot and dry. A balance of these humors was necessary to maintain health (Reinert, 1986; Rose, 1978).

The hot-cold dichotomy was also used as a health classification system. Thus, diseases, remedies, foods, body organs, and air were categorized as either hot or cold (unrelated to temperature). Consequently health maintenance was dependent on a balance between hot and cold factors (Richardson, 1982). In addition, some Mexican Americans conceptualized health as harmonious relations with both the social and spiritual realms. Therefore, any disruption in social relations or any behaviors that conflicted with cultural norms could be detrimental to health (Harwood, 1981).

Traditional Mexican Americans have believed that illness results from some imbalance or disharmony in the body and/or affairs, and the severity of the disease depends on the degree of imbalance (Reinert, 1986). It has been believed that the causative factors of illness could be either natural (*males naturales*) or witchcraft and supernatural (*mal puesto*). Witchcraft illnesses are caused by the power of a sorcerer (*brujo*) or witch (*bruja*) and can be cured by a religious folk healer (*curandero*). Four of the most common clinical syndromes noted among Mexican Americans are *caida de la mollera, empacho, mal de ojo*, and *susto* (Harwood, 1981; Kuipers, 1991; Reinert, 1986; Stenger-Castro, 1978).

Caida de la mollera (fallen fontanelle) occurs in infants when the parietal or frontal bone of the cranium falls, leaving a "soft spot," which may vibrate during breathing. Traditionally it has been thought to be caused by dropping the baby or by roughly removing the nipple from a nursing infant's mouth. Symptoms include diarrhea, restlessness, fever, and an inability to suck. Folk treatment includes prayers, pushing up on the palate from the inside of the baby's mouth, applying eggs or warm olive oil to the scalp, or holding the infant upside down over a pan of tepid water. Usually the cause of this condition is depression of the fontanelle related to severe dehydration resulting from infant diarrhea (Harwood, 1981). The medical treatment includes intravenous solutions to correct the fluid and electrolyte imbalance (Reinert, 1986).

Empacho ("surfeit," indigestion infection, or blocked intestine) may affect anyone, but generally children and postpartum women are at highest risk (Poteet, 1986). It has been believed to be a dysfunction of the digestive system, caused by a bolus of food that becomes lodged in the intestinal tract. Consumption of certain foods such as eggs, cheese, bananas, and excess white bread are thought to precipitate this disorder. Symptoms include nausea and vomiting, bloating, anorexia, thirst, fever, "gas pains," and crying. Folk treatment involves abdominal massage and taking herbal laxatives. Laxatives may be used routinely to cleanse the gastrointestinal tract and prevent *empacho*, a practice that can lead to laxative abuse and bowel malfunction. *Empacho* is sometimes professionally diagnosed as a serious pathological condition (Harwood, 1981; Reinert, 1986).

Mal de ojo (evil eye) may affect anyone, but pregnant women and young children are thought to be most susceptible. It is believed that a strong person with *vista fuerte* (strong vision) can cause illness by gazing admiringly or enviously at a weaker person. The vague symptoms of this disorder include nervousness, aches and pains, headaches, crying, and fever. The simplest treatment is to have the individual with the evil eye power touch the afflicted person, for this is believed to break the bond of evil (Harwood, 1981; Reinert, 1986).

Susto ("fright sickness") affects individuals of all ages. The condition has been believed to be caused by a frightening or traumatic emotional experience. Symptoms include anexoria, nausea, weight loss, general listlessness, and vertigo. Folk treatment consists of prayers, herbal body massage, and drinking herbal teas (Harwood, 1981; Reinert, 1986).

Folk Practitioners

Curanderos are religious folk healers who believe that their powers come from God. They attempt to correct imbalances by the use of prayers and pledges (*mandas*) to religious saints or to supernatural forces, employing candles and artifacts. *Yerberos* are herbalists who use home remedies in the form of herbs and special diets. *Sobadoras* (*sovadors*) are masseuses who massage and/or manipulate the skeletal system to correct musculoskeletal imbalances. *Albolarios* (witch doctors) specialize in the curing of diseases related to witchcraft. *Parteras* are midwives (Reinert, 1986; Samora, 1978).

Martaus (1986), a community health nurse, studied health-seeking behaviors of Mexican-American migrant farmworkers. She found that the typical behavioral process related to the hot-cold illness model evolved in the following sequence: (1) bed rest, (2) taking aspirin, (3) using home remedies, (4) consulting family and the lay referral network, (5) consulting a folk practitioner, and finally (6) seeing a medical professional.

CULTURAL DIETARY PATTERNS

Mexican food, like that of all Latin American countries, is highly seasoned and spicy. Corn and beans are favorite items. Corn is often softened and ground into meal. Beans are eaten boiled, mashed, and fried. Some popular Mexican dishes include the following:

- *Atole*, a cornmeal gruel.
- *Chile con carne*, beef with garlic seasonings, beans, chili peppers, and sauce.
- *Tortilla*, a thin pancake made of cornmeal and flour, cooked on an ungreased griddle. It is the main food of the poor people. Tortillas can be eaten plain or as part of a *taco* or *enchilada*.
- *Taco*, a tortilla filled with seasoned ground meat, lettuce, plus optional ingredients, and served with chili sauce.
- *Enchilada*, a tortilla rolled with sauce, cheese, onion, and shredded lettuce.

- *Sopaipillas*, puffs of deep-fried dough, usually served with honey and eaten as bread or dessert.
- *Tamales*, seasoned ground meat on *masa* (dried ground corn), wrapped in corn husks, then steamed and served with chili sauce (Ensminger, Ensminger, Kolande & Robson, 1983).

There are apparently no special food taboos for Mexican-American Roman Catholics. Pope John XXIII lifted the ban on eating meat on Friday (Ensminger et al., 1983).

MORBIDITY AND MORTALITY

Mexican Americans exhibit a high incidence of diabetes mellitus. Findings indicate that the prevalence of diabetes type II (noninsulin dependent) is 36% higher among Mexican Americans in San Antonio than Mexicans in Mexico (Stern, Gonzalez, Mitchell, Villalpando, Haffner & Hazuda, 1992). This high incidence is apparently associated with an unfavorable distribution of body fat (Haffner, Mitchell, Stern, Hazuda & Patterson, 1992). Of the Hispanic groups, a relatively low incidence of diabetes was found among Cubans as compared to a relatively high incidence among Mexican Americans and Puerto Ricans. These differences may be related to genetic, behavioral, socioeconomic, or environmental factors (Flegal, Ezzati, Harris, Haynes, Juarez & Knowler, 1991).

Obesity is a risk factor for major chronic diseases such as hypertension, heart disease, and cancers of the breast and colon. Thirty-nine percent of Mexican-American women are estimated to be overweight, and 16% of these women are severely overweight or obese. These data were obtained from the Hispanic Health and Nutrition Examination Survey (1982–1984), which included 1,782 Mexican-American, 479 Cuban-American, and 750 Puerto Rican women aged 25 to 74 (Lopez & Masse, 1992).

Cysticercosis or intestinal tapeworm disease appears to occur at a high incidence among Mexican-American immigrants. Some cases were found to be travel related (6.5%) and occurred in persons born in the United States who had traveled to Mexico. Cysticercosis causes notable morbidity and mortality in Los Angeles County. Public health professionals diagnose and treat carriers of the *Taenia* tapeworm (Sorvillo, Waterman, Richards & Schantz, 1992).

Systolic blood pressure was found to be lowest among Mexican Americans when compared to Anglos and African Americans. Mexican-American girls showed a tendency toward less impatience and aggression than the other groups. Mexican Americans had relatively low heart rates (Higginbotham, Baranowski, Puhl & Greaves, 1991).

A high incidence of drug-resistant tuberculosis exists among Mexican Americans in south Texas, of whom 6% are homeless. A high incidence of drug-resistant tuberculosis also exists among the homeless of various cultures in New York (Morris & McAllister, 1992).

Of three Hispanic groups studied (Cuban Americans, Mexican Americans, and Puerto Ricans), Mexican Americans had a death rate intermediate between the other two cultures for all causes of illness. Of the three, Mexican Americans had the highest death rate for cerebrovascular diseases and a high rate (similar to Puerto Ricans) for diabetes mellitus. Mexican Americans had the lowest suicide rate of the other Hispanics and Anglos (Rosenwaike, 1987).

BELIEFS ABOUT DEATH AND DYING

Some Mexican Americans hold concepts of death and dying that are rooted in Roman Catholicism. Religious practices such as saying the rosary (a series of prayers) for the dead are integral parts of mourning. Some view death and hardship as God's will. Expressions of grief tend to be demonstrative. Somatic complaints often reflect the emotional imbalance of grief (Lawson, 1990).

Many Mexican Americans demonstrate their respect for the concept of death through their art, songs, literature, and daily rituals. Death may be viewed as respectful or humorous. This dual-nature concept of death is manifested in celebrations of the annual Day of the Dead, which honors the dead but humorously teases the living about their eventual fate (Villarruel & de Montellano, 1992).

PHYSICAL ASSESSMENT

Compared to non-Hispanic white individuals, Mexican Americans may be shorter. They may have shorter legs but longer trunks. Body fat and fat distribution tend to differ with socioeconomic status and level of acculturation (Lopez & Masse, 1992).

REFERENCES

Allen, J. P., & Turner, E. J. (1988). *We the people: Atlas of American ethnic diversity.* New York: Macmillan.

Becerra, R. M. (1988). The Mexican American family. In C. H. Mindel, R. W. Haberstein & R. Wright, Jr. (Eds.), *Ethnic families in America: Patterns and variations* (3d Ed.) (pp. 141–59). New York: Elsevier.

Bullough, V. L., & Bullough, B. (1982). *Health care for the other Americans.* New York: Appleton-Century-Crofts.

Bureau of the Census. (1988, 1992). *Statistical abstract of the United States.* Washington, DC: Government Printing Office.

Daniels, R. (1990). *Coming to America: A history of immigration and ethnicity in American life.* Princeton, NJ: HarperCollins.

Ensminger, A. H., Ensminger, M. E., Kolande, J. E., & Robson, R. K. (1983). *Diets of the world.* Clovis, CA: Pegus Press.

Falicov, C. J. (1982). Mexican families. In M. McGoldrick, J. K. Pearce & J. Giordano (Eds.), *Ethnicity and family therapy* (pp. 134–63). New York: Guilford Press.

Flegal, K. M., Ezzati, T. M., Harris, M. I., Haynes, S. G., Juarez, R. Z., Knowler, W. C.,

Perez-Stable, E. G., & Stern, M. P. (1991). Prevalence of diabetes in Mexican Americans, Cubans, and Puerto Ricans from the Hispanic Health and Nutrition Examination Survey, 1982–1984. *Diabetes Care, 14*(7), 628–38.

Griswold del Castillo, R. (1984). *La Familia: Chicano families in the urban Southwest, 1848 to present.* Notre Dame: University of Notre Dame Press.

Haffner, S. M., Mitchell, B. D., Stern, M. P., Hazuda, H. P., & Patterson, J. K. (1992). Public health significance of upper body adiposity for non–insulin dependent diabetes mellitus in Mexican Americans. *International Journal of Obesity, 16*(3), 177–84.

Harwood, A. (1981). *Ethnicity and medical care.* Cambridge: Harvard University Press.

Higginbotham, J. C., Baranowski, T., Puhl, J., & Greaves, K. A. (1991). Ethnicity, gender, and type A differences in resting heart rate and blood pressure among young children. *Ethn. Dis. 1*(2), 123–34.

Kuipers, J. (1991). Mexican Americans. In J. N. Giger & R. E. Davidhizar (Eds.), *Transcultural nursing: Assessment and intervention* (pp. 185–212). St. Louis: Mosby Year Book.

Lawson, L. V. (1990, March–April). Culturally sensitive support for grieving parents. *American Journal of Maternal Child Nursing, 15*, 76–79.

Levine, E. S., & Padilla, A. M. (1980). *Crossing cultures in therapy*, Belmont, CA: Wadsworth.

Lopez, L. M., & Masse, B. (1992). Comparison of body mass indexes and cutoff points for estimating the prevalence of overweight in Hispanic women. *Journal of the American Dietetic Association, 92*(11), 1343–47.

McKenzie, T. L., Sallis, J. F., Nader, P. R., Broyles, S. L., & Nelson, J. A. (1992). Anglo and Mexican-American preschoolers at home and at recess: Activity patterns and environmental influences. *Journal of Developmental and Behavioral Pediatrics, 13*(3), 173–80.

Martaus, T. M. (1986). The health-seeking process of Mexican American migrant farmworkers. *Home Health Care Nurse, 4*(5), 32–38.

Monrroy, L.S.A. (1983). Nursing care of Raza/Latino patients. In M. S. Orque, B. Bloch & L.S.A. Monrroy (Eds.), *Ethnic nursing care: A multicultural approach* (pp. 115–48). St. Louis: C. V. Mosby.

Morris, J. T., & McAllister, C. K. (1992). Homeless individuals and drug-resistant tuberculosis in south Texas. *Chest, 102*(3), 802–4.

Murillo, N. (1978). The Mexican American family. In R. A. Martinez (Ed.), *Hispanic culture and health care: Fact, fiction, folklore* (pp. 3–18). St. Louis: C. V. Mosby Co.

Poteet, G. W. (1986). Ethnic diversity. *Journal of Nursing Administration, 16*(3), 6.

Reinert, B. R. (1986). The health care beliefs and values of Mexican-Americans. *Home Health Care Nurse, 4*(5), 23, 26–27, 30–31.

Richardson, L. (1982). Caring through understanding: Part 2, Folk medicine in the Hispanic population. *Imprint, 29*(2), 29–31.

Rose, L. C. (1978). *Disease beliefs in Mexican-American communities.* San Francisco: R & E Research Associates.

Rosenwaike, I. (1987). Mortality differentials among persons born in Cuba, Mexico, and Puerto Rico residing in the United States, 1979–1982. *American Journal of Public Health, 77*(5), 603–6.

Rudolph, J. D. (1985). *Mexico: A country study* (3rd Ed.). Washington, DC: American University.

Samora, A. J. (1978). Conceptions of health and disease among Spanish-Americans. In R. A. Martinez (Ed.), *Hispanic culture and health care: Fact, fiction, folklore* (pp. 65–74). St. Louis: C. V. Mosby Co.

Sorvillo, F. J., Waterman, S. H., Richards, F. O., & Schantz, P. M. (1992). Cysticercosis surveillance: Locally acquired and travel-related infections of intestinal tapeworm carriers in Los Angeles County. *American Journal of Tropical Medicine and Hygiene, 47*(3), 365–71.

Stenger-Castro, E. M. (1978). The Mexican-American: How his culture affects his mental health. In R. A. Martinez (Ed.), *Hispanic culture and health care: Fact, fiction, folklore* (pp. 19–32). St. Louis: C. V. Mosby Co.

Stern, M. P., Gonzalez, C., Mitchell, B. D., Villalpando, E., Haffner, S. M., & Hazuda, H. P. (1992). Genetic and environmental determinants of type II diabetes in Mexico City and San Antonio. *Diabetes, 41*(4), 484–92.

Valdez, A. (1980). *Ethnic maintenance among Mexicans and Puerto Ricans.* Report to Southwestern Sociological Association.

Villarruel, A. M., & de Montellano, B. O. (1992). Culture and pain: A Mesoamerican perspective. *Advances in Nursing Science, 15*(1), 21–32.

15

Vietnamese Americans

The countries of Vietnam, Laos, and Cambodia (Kampuchea) are often referred to as Indochina or Southeast Asia. Vietnam, situated on the eastern coast of the Indochinese peninsula, is bordered on the north by China and on the south by the Gulf of Thailand. Cambodia and Laos border Vietnam on the west, while the South China Sea forms the eastern border. Vietnam occupies an area slightly smaller than Japan.

Historically, the Vietnamese people have been dominated by foreign invaders. The Chinese dominated Vietnam for 1,000 years, and later the French colonized the country for 100 years. After the French colonization, civil war erupted, and North and South Vietnam fought each other (Tran, 1988). In 1954 the Geneva Accords divided Vietnam into the Communist north and non-Communist south. Conflicts between the Soviet-assisted North Vietnam and the U.S.-assisted South Vietnam ended in 1975, and Vietnam was reunited as the Republic of North Vietnam.

Vietnam is a tropical country. Although the northern areas have four distinct seasons, the southern portions have only a rainy and dry season.

POPULATION IN THE UNITED STATES

Vietnamese Americans number 615,000, representing 0.2% of the U.S. population. Fifty-four percent of the Vietnamese Americans reside in the West, and 20% reside in the South (Bureau of the Census, 1992). The largest numbers of this population are found in California, Virginia, Texas, and Florida (Lan, 1988). California is the Vietnamese capital in the United States. California Vietnamese

Americans control the Vietnamese market in America; they publish Vietnamese books and produce Vietnamese videos, movies, and food for their population in America and throughout the rest of the world (Tran, 1988). Over 90% of Vietnamese Americans were born in Vietnam (Bureau of the Census, 1992), and generally they tend to be a young population when compared to other immigrant groups in the United States.

IMMIGRATION

In 1975 when the South Vietnamese government collapsed, there was a major exodus from South Vietnam to avoid persecution by the North Vietnamese Communists. This first wave of Vietnamese immigrants consisted mainly of professionals, government officials, military personnel, and religious leaders, many of them affiliated with the United States and the collapsed Thieu regime. These first South Vietnamese refugees were for the most part well educated (more than 25% college graduates), young (88% younger than 45 years of age), Catholic (55%), and in good health; most arrived in family groups (62% in families of at least five persons). This group largely adapted successfully to American society (Montero, 1979; Stauffer, 1991; Tran, 1988).

In contrast, many refugees of the second wave were not as well educated, less familiar with Western life-style, less healthy, and less able to speak English than the first wave. They were often called "boat people" because many emerged by boat to Thailand, Malaysia, Singapore, or Japan (Muecke, 1983; Tran, 1988). Escape attempts were typically long, hazardous, and often fatal for up to 50% of the escapees. Many spent as many as seven years in Southeast Asian camps in desperate circumstances. By the time they arrived in the United States, they had been separated from their families and had experienced severe physical and emotional trauma (Muecke, 1983). Those who migrated often faced abrupt termination of familial and peer attachments and found few formal educational opportunities in their native language. In addition, the absence of an ethnic enclave in the new community often further deprived the new immigrant of a support system (Fabrega & Nguyen, 1992).

COMMUNICATION

Vietnamese is the language of most individuals from Vietnam. Before the 1960s, educated Vietnamese persons also spoke French. By 1975, English had become the more popular second language. Some Vietnamese-Chinese speak Chinese. There are three distinct dialects of the Vietnamese language, characteristic of the northern, central, and southern regions of Vietnam.

The word *yes* in English expresses agreement; however, *ya* for a Vietnamese may indicate respect and not necessarily agreement. The polite *ya, ya* ("*Ya, ya, Thua Ba, ya ya*") may be interpreted by an American to mean, "Yes, yes, I'll do it," whereas the Vietnamese American may mean, "I'm listening, and I respect what you are saying.'' This lack of mutual understanding could be problematic in verbal communication between American health professionals and Vietnamese-American clients. The health professional's perception of noncompliance by some Vietnamese Americans could be related to this misinterpretation of *ya* (Stauffer, 1991).

Some Vietnamese Americans may avoid eye contact when talking to a person viewed as a superior. This is a way of showing respect. A person likely to be considered superior is someone with more education, or of a higher social status, or older.

Vietnamese Americans tend to prefer more personal space during social relationships than that desired by many persons of mainstream American culture. Some Vietnamese Americans may consider the head a sacred part of the body. Therefore it might not be appropriate to pat the head during communication (Stauffer, 1991).

SOCIOECONOMIC STATUS

In general the average income of Vietnamese Americans is lower than that of most other American families. Income is positively related to English-speaking ability (Portes & Rumbaut, 1990). Many Vietnamese Americans place a high value on education and have made great strides in this area. As of 1988, at least 8% of all Vietnamese-American women and 18% of the men over 25 years of age had college educations (Bureau of the Census, 1988). In addition, at least 27% of Vietnamese Americans are home owners. This manifests an admirable elevation of socioeconomic status considering the fact that most Vietnamese have been in this country for less than 20 years (Stauffer, 1991).

CHIEF COMPLAINT

Negative emotions are rarely expressed in public. An exception may be the expected wailing of a widow at the death of her husband. Vietnamese Americans place a high value on self-control in speech and behavior. Somatization is frequently noted among Vietnamese Americans, perhaps related to the suppression of negative emotions and thus the expression through various physical ailments (Stauffer, 1991). Vietnamese Americans tend to be stoic and noncomplaining. An expectation that nature will cure and a fear of invasive procedures may cause this individual to postpone seeking care for a blatant pathologic disorder (Muecke, 1983; Stauffer, 1991).

FAMILY

The Traditional Family

To the Vietnamese American, the family is a social entity that consists of all one's relatives—not just father, mother, and siblings but an extended unit. Each member cares more about family than self. The traditional Vietnamese family is similar to the traditional Chinese family in terms of its ethical and moral structure (Vuong, 1976; Che, 1979).

The traditional kinship system has been patrilineal, or male oriented (Luong, 1984). Family loyalty focuses on filial piety, which emphasizes that children should honor and obey their parents. This obligation extends even after the parents' death, when children commemorate their parents and care for their graves (Tran, 1988).

The Vietnamese-American term for kinship system is *Ho*, which denotes an extended family including both living and dead members. Two types of *Ho* are *Ho Noi*, composed of all relatives on the father's side, and *Ho Ngoai*, consisting of all relatives on the mother's side. Members of the *Ho Noi* are forbidden to intermarry, but third-generation *Ho Ngoai* can intermarry (Luong, 1984). Traditionally, the oldest male (*Truong Toc*) is the head of the family. The *Truong Toc* is responsible for maintaining the family land and ancestral graves and perpetuating ancestor worship. The heads of the traditional Vietnamese nuclear family are often the grandparents. At their deaths the father becomes the head, to be succeeded by his son. The head of the family completely controls his family and even assumes responsibility for the behavior of individual members. He is legally accountable for failing to prevent any member of his family from committing a crime (Tran, 1988).

Traditional Vietnamese women have had no power and few privileges. A woman is expected to honor and obey the father, then her husband, and finally her eldest son, with whom she will live when she is a widow. However, the traditional Vietnamese woman gains status when she becomes a mother because she then ranks second in the family after the father (Tran, 1988).

The Modern Family

Many of the traditional values are still held by many Vietnamese Americans. However, the American economic system has necessitated some changes. Vietnamese-American children tend to become more economically independent. Many children quickly become more knowledgeable about American society than their parents and demand more freedom than tradition has allowed. Many young Vietnamese, having moved away from their families to pursue educational and professional opportunities, were unable to maintain the traditional practice of living with their parents until marriage. The modern Vietnamese-American father has lost some of his absolute power over the family. His children often react differently because they are becoming acculturated to a different culture. The father finds that methods of punishment used in Vietnam may be inappropriate in America (Tran, 1988).

Due to economic necessity, the Vietnamese-American woman may obtain a job outside the home. Working and contributing to the family support gives her increased status and power in the family, although the husband usually remains the dominant authority figure. Vietnamese Americans were found to be the only Asian group with a relatively high percentage (14.2%) of households headed by women (Gardner, Robey & Smith, 1985).

A study by Kibria (1990) explored the effect of migration on gender roles of Vietnamese men and women. Ethnographic interviews were conducted with 15 men and 16 women from a community of recently settled Vietnamese immigrants in the United States. The women played important roles as mediators in family disputes and in the distribution of economic resources among households. These activities allowed women an accepted informal power that buffered male authority in the family. However, despite their increased power and economic resources, these women strongly supported a patriarchal social structure because they felt that it preserved parental authority and promoted greater future economic security for the family.

ELDERLY

Traditionally Vietnamese elderly were powerful and highly respected for their wisdom. However, the traditional wisdom that could be passed down is less useful in American society. Therefore, Vietnamese-American elderly have lost a great deal of their power. Since many do not speak English and cannot drive, they are often highly dependent on yet often isolated from their families. Their grandchildren often prefer to speak English and watch American television. In many Vietnamese-American communities, the elderly experience loneliness and homesickness for the homeland. Often their only social outlet is the church (Tran, 1988).

CHILD REARING

Vietnamese-American women have a significantly higher fertility rate than all other major Asian-American women: Chinese, Japanese, Filipino, Korean, and Asian Indian (Stauffer, 1991; Tran, 1988). Data from San Francisco and San Diego indicate that the Vietnamese-American fertility rate has been high since their arrival in the United States. Fertility rates were found to be significantly higher among rural second-wave refugees than in the more urban first-wave groups. Families often exceeded five children per mother, as was the practice in the homeland. The data suggest that this refugee population will continue to use American maternal and child health resources heavily, but that residence in the United States might eventually motivate desires to limit family size (Rumbaut, Brindis, Korenbrot & Minkler, 1989). Before admission to the United States, most Vietnamese mothers were unfamiliar with birth control methods because of their perceived need for large families to replace those lost to war, starvation, and illness. When birth control was addressed by American health professionals, about 80% of the Vietnamese refugees chose some method of contraception (Sutherland, Avant, Franz, Monzon & Stark, 1983).

Some Vietnamese-American children have expressed a sense of being torn between two cultures. For example, the American practice of teenage dating has been prohibited in traditional Vietnamese society, where parents exercise greater control than do American parents. There is a significant generation gap because many of the Vietnamese who migrated in 1975 still uphold the old traditions and the youth have acculturated more rapidly than their parents. Some second-generation Vietnamese-American youths enjoy the new freedom and have joined gangs in a quest for more freedom and to rebel against the traditional ways (Cowell, 1993).

Displaced Amerasian youths—children of Vietnamese mothers and American fathers—were found to be particularly susceptible to street gang affiliation. Many of these Amerasian children, with no father figure, experienced a sense of abandonment and consequently turned to the belongingness of street gangs. The organization Friends of Amerasian Children has many volunteers who work diligently to locate fathers of Vietnamese youth and unite families (Padgett, 1990).

SOCIALIZATION PATTERNS

A distinct characteristic of Vietnamese culture is an emphasis on moderation and caution. Children are taught to think before speaking. Modesty of action and speech are stressed. A slip of the tongue could disrupt harmony in a relationship. Many Vietnamese Americans believe that "bragging reflects an empty soul." Overt expression of emotions is considered in bad taste except in selected private situations. Emotions may be viewed as signs of weakness because they interfere with self-control. Romantic expressions and gestures are usually reserved for private situations. Public displays of joy and happiness are rarely practiced by most Vietnamese Americans. An exception to the usual restraint may be the expected wailing and demonstrative behavior of a widow on the death of her husband (Stauffer, 1991). The cultural background of the Vietnamese emphasizes premarital virginity and modesty (Sutherland et al., 1983).

Vietnamese Americans have a popular saying, "Suspicious as Tao Thao." Ta Thao was a well-known, very suspicious, and successful Chinese politician. The statement implies that a highly suspicious person is not necessarily paranoid. Instead this person has a heightened social awareness of self manifested by an emphasis on moral and social obligations. This person is concerned with group harmony and is sensitive to the feelings and rights of others in social settings. A demeanor of suspicion, distrust, alienation, and anticipated victimization or a paranoid outlook is sometimes found in Vietnamese immigrants who are acculturating slowly or feel alienated from American society (Mirowsky & Ross, 1983; Portes & Rumbaut, 1990).

RELIGIOUS BELIEFS AND PRACTICES

Many religions have influenced the Vietnamese-American belief system. The most influential are Buddhism, Confucianism, and Taoism. Buddhist principles, which encompass a belief in reincarnation and that life is suffering, have significantly influenced the Vietnamese characteristics of stoicism, self-control, and apparent passivity (Fabrega & Nguyen, 1992; Stauffer, 1991). Some Vietnamese adhere to animism, a belief in supernatural forces and spiritualism (Lawson, 1990). (See Chapter 3, on Chinese Americans, for a discussion of Confucianism and Taoism.)

A number of Vietnamese Americans are Roman Catholic. When Pope John Paul II visited Denver in August 1993, he singled out the Vietnamese Americans as the only ethnic group with whom he would meet. Vietnamese church leaders said that the pope extended this privilege partially because as a Pole who felt suppressed in a Communist nation, he felt a particular affinity for the Vietnamese people because he could identify with their suffering (Cowell, 1993).

CULTURALLY BASED HEALTH BELIEFS AND PRACTICES

Traditionally, Vietnamese Americans have a holistic concept of health—a belief that health is dependent on family, religion, food, morality, and metaphysical forces (Sutherland et al., 1983). Some Vietnamese Americans believe in several causes of illness: supernatural, metaphysical, or germ related (Stauffer, 1991).

The natural theory is similar to the Hippocratic concept based on the healing power of nature. Hippocratic principles view the person as composed of bodily humors in a natural environment. The healthy person is in harmony with his or her environment. Diagnosis in this framework involves observation of the client's physical and social environment. Treatment consists of promoting the client's natural recuperative powers. Massage, tonics, and avoidance of excesses are common natural health maintenance behaviors for some Vietnamese Americans (Muecke, 1983).

Supernatural diseases are caused by supernatural powers such as gods, demons, or spirits. Some believe that spirits and deities frequently interfere in a person's life activities. Thus, sometimes an individual may sense the presence of someone who is not visible in the environment. Although these perceptual experiences may appear pathological in Western societies, they are not necessarily viewed as such by many Vietnamese Americans (Fabrega & Nguyen, 1992; Stauffer, 1991).

The metaphysical theory is based on a balance of hot and cold, or yin and yang (Muecke, 1983; Stauffer, 1991), which is discussed at length in Chapter 3 on Chinese Americans.

Some Vietnamese postpartum women may refuse to take baths, wash their heads, or drink juices or water for fear of upsetting the "hot" and "cold" balance in their bodies. Because some consider blood the fire element, its loss after delivery could put the body at risk for becoming too cold. Consequently activities that chill the body are avoided. Wadd (1983) interviewed 20 Vietnamese families in Salt Lake City, Utah, and found that special diets and activity regimes were widely practiced by primipara but less rigidly by multipara mothers. Suggested postpartum activities included the avoidance of cold, including drafts and showers, and the avoidance of sexual intercourse. Limited activity and bed rest were also important practices.

Similarly, some Vietnamese Americans prefer to treat a fever by dressing the febrile person warmly and restricting fluids, fruits, and vegetables. Again the underlying theory is that since the body is already losing too much heat, foods classified as cold, such as fruits and vegetables, should be avoided. Instead they prefer to substitute neutral foods such as rice, eggs, sweets, chicken broth, and teas. The hot-cold belief system is evident in the self-care behaviors of many Vietnamese Americans regardless of educational level (Muecke, 1983; Stauffer, 1991). Some believe that Western medications are generally hot and very potent. Although many Vietnamese clients expect to receive a prescription when visiting a physician, the client may decrease the dosage to prevent untoward effects or discontinue the medication if symptoms are not relieved within a few days (Tung, 1980).

Dermabrasive procedures represent another group of self-care practices noted among some Vietnamese Americans. These procedures are used to alleviate a wide variety of symptoms such as headache, nausea, myalgia, cough, and backache. The procedures abrade the skin with minor scrapes that are rarely harmful but help the person experience a sense of control over the problem. A cutaneous hematoma is sometimes created over an affected area of the face, neck, chest, or back to release excessive "air" believed to cause certain conditions. There are various methods used to induce hematomas: by pinching the skin; by rubbing an oiled skin with the edge of a coin, spoon, or piece of bamboo; or by placing a cup from which oxygen has been extracted through heating over the affected area for 15 to 30 minutes (giac cup suction). If the client is a child, the health professional should be cautious not to confuse this evidence of home treatment with evidence of child abuse (Golden & Duster, 1977; Muecke, 1983; Yeatman & Dang, 1980; Stauffer, 1991).

CULTURAL DIETARY PATTERNS

Vietnamese-American food reflects Chinese and French influences. The common staple of the Vietnamese diet is rice. A salty fish paste or sauce is added to many dishes for flavor (Tran, 1990). Rice and other dishes are seasoned with this sauce (nuoc nam), made by marinating small fish in salt for a month or more. Meat cut into small pieces may be eaten with rice and vegetables. Bean curd is another favorite, although dry bean dishes are not common (Stauffer, 1991). Lemon-beef salad and shrimp crepes are favorites (Tran, 1990).

The traditional Vietnamese diet is low in fat and sugar, moderate in fiber, and high in complex carbohydrates (Burtis, Davis & Martin, 1988). Although tea is considered the favorite drink, many Vietnamese Americans enjoy water and soft drinks. Before migration, Vietnamese were not great fluid drinkers, a practice that has been related to bladder stones in males. Also, since many Vietnamese Americans have a lactose intolerance, milk was seldom included in their diet (Hoang & Erickson, 1982).

Strict Buddhists are vegetarians. Many avoid eating the flesh of any animal and may not eat eggs or drink milk. They will eat fish because fish are merely removed from the water, not slaughtered. Many strict Buddhists abstain from intoxicating beverages (Ensminger, Ensminger, Kolande & Robson, 1983).

MORBIDITY AND MORTALITY

Reizian and Meleis (1987) studied and compared symptoms reported by Arab Americans, Vietnamese Americans, native-born Americans, and other cultural groups at the University of Oregon Medical School Hospital. Arab Americans and Vietnamese Americans reported the highest number of symptoms pertaining to the digestive system, and both groups demonstrated similarly high psychological symptom patterns for feelings of inadequacy. Feelings of tension were noted as the second most common psychological symptom for Vietnamese Americans. Generally the Vietnamese Americans reported slightly more psychological symptoms than the Arab Americans. Also Vietnamese Americans reported more symptoms related to the respiratory and nervous systems than the Arab Americans.

A significant number of Vietnamese Americans have been diagnosed as having psychiatric or psychosomatic problems. A high prevalence of depression exists among the second-wave refugee groups as determined by the Vietnamese Depression Rating Scale, which was developed for testing this group (Sutherland, Avant & Franz, 1983). Although the origins of some emotional responses and illnesses of Vietnamese migrants may be unrelated to traumatic events, refugee trauma increases the likelihood of certain emotional responses, such as anxiety, depression, delayed grief, and posttraumatic stress disorder (Muecke, 1983).

Sutherland et al. (1983) studied the health status of 426 Indochinese refugees, of whom 208 were Vietnamese. Findings indicated that this was a young population that was generally very healthy. Prevalent infectious diseases included intestinal parasites, tuberculosis, and hepatitis B. Thirty-five percent of these refugees manifested hematologic abnormalities, mainly microcytosis. As compared to the other two study groups (Laotians and Cambodians), the Vietnamese had the lowest rate of anemia and microcytosis. Results of an earlier study (Monzon, Fairbanks, Burgert & Elliot, 1981) found that thalassemias and hemoglobin E trait are the most common causes of microcytosis in Southeast Asians. Microcytosis may be incorrectly diagnosed as anemia and consequently inappropriately treated with iron. Therefore physicians should be aware that erythrocytic microcytosis in Southeast Asians is most likely a reflection of the presence of thalassemia or of hemoglobin E trait (Luan, 1969). These conditions are usually harmless and do not require treatment (Sutherland et al., 1983).

Results of a study by Chung and Kagawa-Singer (1993) indicated that Vietnamese women were more likely to experience distress than their husbands. They also found that regardless of the number of years in the United States, premigration trauma events and refugee camp experiences served as significant predictors of psychological distress for up to five years after migration. Results of another study (Buchwald, Manson, Dinges, Keane & Kinzie, 1993) also noted the prevalence of depressive symptoms among Vietnamese Americans. Although physical symptoms that created anxiety about health status existed, psychological and emotional symptoms were much more prevalent. However, Ganesan, Fine, and Lin (1989) observed that Vietnamese Americans tend to refuse mental health services until symptoms are severe.

BELIEFS ABOUT DEATH AND DYING

Generally major beliefs are related to religious affiliation. Some Vietnamese Americans believe in the constant presence of ancestors' spirits. Buddhists uphold the theory of reincarnation (Fabrega & Nguyen, 1992). Mourning families may wear white clothing or head bands for a certain period of time. Vietnamese generally bury their dead, whereas Cambodians and Laotians tend to prefer cremation. Some Vietnamese Americans may express grief as somatic complaints (Lawson, 1990).

PHYSICAL ASSESSMENT

Vietnamese Americans generally have small body frames and are seldom overweight, except for some Vietnamese-Chinese individuals. Vietnamese skin color is light to medium, with yellow tones. Eyelids have an epicanthic fold, noses may be small, and teeth may be proportionately large. These characteristics are typical of Asian individuals (Stauffer, 1991; Williams & Westermeyer, 1986).

REFERENCES

Buchwald, D., Manson, S. M., Dinges, N. G., Keane, E. M., & Kinzie, J. D. (1993). Prevalence of depressive symptoms among established Vietnamese refugees in the United States: Detection in a primary care setting. *Journal of General Internal Medicine, 8*(2), 76–81.

Bureau of the Census. (1988, 1992). *Statistical abstracts of the United States.* Washington, DC: Government Printing Office.

Burtis, G., Davis, J., & Martin, S. (1988). *Applied nutrition and diet therapy.* Philadelphia: W. B. Saunders Co.

Che, W. (1979). *The modern Chinese family.* Palo Alto, CA: R & E Research Associates.

Cowell, A. (1993, August 15). Vietnamese identity split, wait for pope. *New York Times,* p. 12.

Chung, R. C., Kagawa-Singer, M. (1993). Predictors of psychological distress among southeast Asian refugees. *Social Science and Medicine, 36*(5), 631–39.

Ensminger, A. H., Ensminger, M. E., Kolande, J. E., & Robson, R. K. (1983). *Foods and nutrition encyclopedia* (Vol. 1). Clovis, CA: Pegus Press.

Fabrega, H., Jr., & Nguyen, H. (1992, August). Culture, social structure, and quandaries of psychiatric diagnosis: A Vietnamese case study. *Psychiatry, 55,* 230–49.

Ganesan, S., Fine, S., & Lin, T. Y. (1989). Psychiatric symptoms in refugee families from South East Asia: Therapeutic challenges. *American Journal of Psychotherapy, 43*(2), 218–28.

Gardner, R. W., Robey, B., & Smith, P. C. (1985). Asian Americans: Growth, change and diversity. *Population Bulletin, 40,* 1–44.

Golden, S. M., & Duster, M. C. (1977). Hazards of misdiagnosis due to Vietnamese folk medicine. *Clinical Pediatrics, 16,* 949–50.

Hoang, G., & Erickson, R. (1982). Guidelines for providing medical care for Southeast Asian refugees. *JAMA, 248*(6), 710–14.

Kibria, N. (1990). Power, patriarchy, and gender conflict in the Vietnamese immigrant community. *Gender and Society, 4*(1), 9–24.

Lan, L. V. (1988). Folk medicine among Southeast Asian refugees in the United States: Risks, benefits and uncertainties. *Journal of the Association of Vietnamese Medical Professionals in Canada, 98,* 31–36.

Lawson, L. V. (1990 March–April). Culturally sensitive support for grieving parents. *MCN, 15,* 76–79.

Luan, L. I. (1969). Distribution of genetic red cell defects in South-east Asia. *Transactions, Royal Society of Tropical Medicine and Hygiene, 63,* 664.

Luong, H. V. (1984). Brother and uncle: An analysis of rules, structures, contradictions and meaning in Vietnamese kinship. *American Anthropologist, 86,* 290–315.

Mirowsky, J., & Ross, C. E. (1983). Paranoia and the structure of powerlessness. *American Sociological Review, 48,* 228–39.

Montero, D. (1979). *Vietnamese Americans: Patterns of resettlement and socioeconomic adaptation in the United States.* Boulder, CO: Westview Press.

Monzon, C. M., Fairbanks, V. F., Burgert, E. O., & Elliot, S. O. (1981). Hematologic and genetic disorders of SE Asian refugees, abstract. *Blood, 48*(Suppl 1), 55a.

Muecke, M. A. (1983). In search of healers: Southeast Asian refugees in the American health care system. *Western Journal of Medicine, 139*(6), 835–40.

Padgett, T. (1990, April 9). Like meeting my dad: Amerasians, vets bond. *Newsweek,* p. 65.

Portes, A., & Rumbaut, R. G. (1990). *Immigrant America.* Berkeley: University of California Press.

Reizian, A., & Meleis, A. I. (1987). Symptoms reported by Arab-American patients on the Cornell Medical Index (CMI). *Western Journal of Nursing Research, 9*(3), 368–84.

Rumbaut, R. G., Brindis, C., Korenbrot, C. C., & Minkler, D. (1989). High fertility among Indochinese refugees. *Public Health Report, 104*(2), 143–50.

Stauffer, R. Y. (1991). Vietnamese Americans. In J. N. Giger & R. E. Davidhizar (Eds.), *Transcultural nursing: Assessment and intervention* (pp. 403–34). St. Louis: Mosby Year Book.

Sutherland, J. E., Avant, R. F., Franz, W. B., Monzon, C. M., & Stark, N. M. (1983). Indoese refugee health assessment and treatment. *Journal of Family Practice, 16*, 61–67.

Tran, P. (1990). *Living and cooking Vietnamese: An American woman's experience.* Corona: Taylor Publishing.

Tran, T. V. (1988). The Vietnamese American family. In C. H. Mindel, R. W. Haberstein & R. Wright, Jr. (Eds.), *Ethnic families in America: Patterns and variations* (3d ed.) (pp. 276–99). New York: Elsevier Science Publishing Co.

Tung, T. M. (1980). Indochinese patients: Cultural aspects of the medical and psychiatric care of Indochinese refugees. *Action for South East Asians*, pp. 13–16, 30–35.

Vuong, G. T. (1976). *Getting to know Vietnamese and their culture.* New York: Ungar.

Wadd, L. (1983). Vietnamese postpartum practices: Implications for nursing in the hospital setting. *JOGN Nursing, 12*(4), 252–58.

Williams, C., & Westermeyer, J. (1986). *Refugee mental health in resettlement countries.* New York: Hemisphere.

Yeatman, G. W., & Dang, V. V. (1980). Cao Gio (coin rubbing) Vietnamese attitudes toward health care. *JAMA, 244*, 2748–49.

Index

Acculturation, xi

African Americans: abnormal color changes, 16; abortions, 5; AIDS, 15; Baptists, 12; Black English, 2; cancer, 14; child rearing, 5–8; diabetes, 14; elderly, 5; family, 3–5; health and illness concepts, natural or unnatural, 8–9; heart disease, 14; herbs, 9; hypertension, 14; Jehovah's Witnesses, 12; lactose intolerance, 11; life expectancy, 13; Methodists, 12; mortality crossover, 5; Muslims/Moslems, 12–13; periodontal disease, 15; philosophy of health, 8; pica, 6; preachers, 11; pregnancy, 5–6; reciprocity, 4; Seventh Day Adventists, 12; sickle cell anemia, 15; sudden infant death syndrome (SIDS), 13

Arab Americans, 21–33; Arab world, 21; Arabic, 22, 31–32; childbirth, 27–28; Christians, 21–22, 25, 28; Egyptians, 22; elderly, 26; evil eye, 27, 30; family, 24–26; intermarriage, 24; Iranians, 22, 23, 30; Islam, 22, 24–26, 29–30; Muslims, 22–23, 25–26, 28–30; Palestinians, 22; pregnancy, 26; Quran, 26, 28–29, 30–31; Ramadan, 30; shame and honor, 29; Syrians, 22; urinary stone disease, 31; veil (*lithma*), 28; Yemenis, 22

Browning of America, xi

Chinese Americans: acupuncture, 43; ancestor worship, 41; Buddhism, 41; childbirth, 39–40; China (PRC), 35; Chinese Pinyin language system, 36, 46–47; Christian religions, 41; Confucianism, 41; elderly, 39; family, 37–39; filial piety, 37; harmony and balance, 40; heart disease, 45; lactose intolerance, 45; Mandarin, 36; neurasthenia, 45; pain, 37; pregnancy, 39; reincarnation, 46; suicide, 40, 46; Taoism, 41; thalassemia, 45; yin and yang, 42

Cuban Americans: cancers, 60; child rearing, 55; cold-hot dichotomy, 57; *compadres*, 55; Cuba, 51; death rate, 59; diabetes, 60; elderly, 54–55; evil eye, 57–58; family, 53–54; health and illness concepts, 57; hypertension, 60;

About the Author

SYBIL M. LASSITER, Associate Professor in Adult and Family/Community Nursing, East Tennessee State University (formerly of Adelphi University, New York), has taught and advised at different institutions in the North and South. Her presentations have emphasized cultural diversity and its impact on the provision of health and social services to America's major ethnic and religious groups. She has also written on the subject in various professional journals.